HEALTH TECH BOOK SERIES

THE MIRACLE CURES OF DIABETES

HOW TO BEAT YOUR DIABETES FOR GOOD!!!

BY

Professor Awad Mansour

**Professor of Chemical & Pharmaceutical
Engineering
Formerly with
University of Akron
OH,U.S.A.**

**First Edition
2011**

HEALTH TECH BOOK SERIES
9923 S.RIDGELAND AVE
SUITE 202
CHICAGO RIDGE IL 60415
U.S.A.

Published and Printed in the United States by:

HEALTH TECH BOOK SERIES

Mansour,Awad

The Miracle Cures of Diabetes

First Edition

ISBN-10: 1463744196
EAN-13: 978-1463744199

HEALTH DISCLAIMER
THE MIRACLE CURES OF DIABETES: IS DESIGNED FOR INFORMATIVE PURPOSES ONLY AND ANY READER IS EXPECTED TO CONSULT HIS FAMILY DOCTOR BEFORE TAKING ANY CHEMICAL OR NATURAL PRODUCTS AND THE AUTHOR IS NOT RESPONSIBLE FOR THE USE OR MISUSE OF THE INFORMATION CONTAINED WITHIN.

TABLE OF CONTENTS

CHAPTER 1
DIABETES CAUSES, SYMPTOMS AND TYPES

Types of Diabetes

There are several different types of diabetes :

Type 1 Diabetes, also known as juvenile or insulin-dependent diabetes which is considered an autoimmune disease, usually develops before age 20 or around it and makes up 5 to 10% of all diabetics. With type 1, the insulin-secreting cells(**BetaCells**) of the pancreas are destroyed partially or totally by the body's immune system as a response to a viral/bacterial infection or some other potentially stressful reasons affecting the body. This results in zero or low percentage of insulin production by the pancreas. This type of diabetes is called **Insulin Dependent(IDM)** since patients need man-made artificial insulin injections in order to be able to burn high sugar in the blood.

Type 2 Diabetes, also known as maturity-onset diabetes, occurs in people older than 40 and makes up 90 to 95% of those with diabetes. With type 2 diabetes, the pancreas may still produce some insulin but not in large enough quantities to properly burn the sugar in the blood stream. This type of diabetes is also called **Insulin Independent Diabetes Mellitus (IIDM)** since Insulin injection is not usually required. Obesity, diet, race, age, lack of exercise, and heredity are all contributing risk factors for type 2 diabetes. Type 2 is most common among Latinos, American Indians, African-Americans and American-Asians.

Gestational Diabetes is another form of type 2 diabetes that develops during pregnancy and affects about 4% of pregnant women. Gestational diabetes is caused by hormonal resistance to insulin. The condition usually disappears after delivery in most women; however, it is a sign that a woman is at a greater risk of developing type 2 diabetes later in life.

Diabetes Insipidus(DI) is a rare form of diabetes usually caused by the deficiency of antidiuretic hormone (ADH) from the pituitary and more rarely by the failure of the kidneys to respond to normal levels of ADH.This condition is characterized by excessive thirst and excretion of large amounts of severely diluted urine, with reduction of fluid intake having no effect on the latter.

Pre-Diabetes is a common condition related to diabetes. In people with pre-diabetes, the blood sugar level is higher than normal but not high enough to be considered diabetic. To make sure that a person is far from diabetes it is essential to measure his/her 3-month accumulated blood sugar average which is known **HbA1c test**.

Pre-diabetes increases the risk of developing type 2 diabetes and of heart disease or stroke. Pre-diabetes can typically be reversed without insulin or medication by losing a reasonable amount of weight and increasing physical activity. This weight loss can prevent, or at least delay, the onset of type 2 diabetes.

According to American Diabetes Association(ADA) about 20% more adults are now believed to have this condition and may develop diabetes within 10 years if they do not exercise or maintain a healthy weight.

About 17 million Americans (6.2% of adults in North America) are believed to have diabetes. About one third of diabetic adults do not know they have diabetes.

About 1 million new cases occur each year, and diabetes is the direct or indirect cause of more than 200,000 deaths each year.

The incidence of diabetes is increasing rapidly. This increase is due to many factors, but the most significant are the obesity and the bad lifestyles.

Symptoms of Diabetes

The symptoms for Type I and Type II diabetes are almost the same and should be immediately investigated by anyone who notices them.

Chapter I

Symptoms of type 1 diabetes include increased thirst, increased hunger, frequent urination, dry mouth, fatigue, unexplained weight loss, eyesight problems and heavy breathing. Loss of consciousness can also occur, but this is very rare.

Symptoms of type 2 diabetes include those listed for type 1 diabetes, plus itchy skin in the vaginal or groin area, yeast infections, slow healing sores, unexplained weight gain, low blood sugar levels, tingling in the extremities and impotence.

We can summarize the symptoms of both types as follows:

Type 1 diabetes symptoms include the following:

- Increased thirst
- Dry mouth
- Increased urination
- Constant hunger
- Unexplained weight loss
- Blurred vision
- Fatigue

Type 2 diabetes symptoms include:

- Very slow healing cuts, scrapes and wounds on the skin
- Nausea
- Recurrent yeast or urinary tract infections
- Increased appetite
- Increased thirst
- Dry mouth
- Frequent urination
- Fatigue/feeling tired
- Unexplained weight loss

- Blurred vision
- Impotence
- Vomiting or diarrhea

Diabetes Causes

Type 1 diabetes: Type 1 diabetes is believed to be an autoimmune disease. The body's immune system attacks the Beta cells that produce insulin in the pancreas.

A predisposition to develop type 1 diabetes may run in families, but genetic factors can not fully explain the development of type 1 diabetes. Environmental factors, including common viral infections, may also contribute. In addition, you may be at risk for type 1 diabetes if you suffer from other hormonal problems such as hypothyroidism or Hashimoto's or Addison's disease.

Type 1 diabetes is caused when certain white blood cells (called T cells) attack and destroy the insulin-producing beta cells in the pancreas. The subsequent lack of insulin leads to increased blood and urine glucose and is fatal unless treated with insulin or alternative herbal formula which can increase the number of beta cells to replace the damaged ones.

Vaccination and Type 1 Diabetes

Vaccines Proven To Be Largest Cause of Insulin Dependent Diabetes in Children

In the May 24, 1996 New Zealand Medical Journal, Dr. Classen reported that there was a 60 percent increase in Type I diabetes (**juvenile diabetes**) following a massive campaign in New Zealand from 1988 to 1991 to vaccinate babies six weeks of age or older with hepatitis B vaccine. His analysis of a group of 100,000 New Zealand children prospectively followed since 1982 showed that the incidence of diabetes before the hepatitis B vaccination program began in 1988 was 11.2 cases per 100,000 children per year while the incidence of diabetes following the hepatitis B vaccination campaign was 18.2 cases per 100,000 children per year. Dr. Classen presented data supporting a causal

Chapter I _____

relationship between many different vaccines and the development of insulin diabetes. The data indicated people with vaccine induced diabetes may not develop the disease until 4 or more years after receiving a vaccine.

Childhood Vaccinations and Juvenile-Onset (Type-1) Diabetes by Harris Coulter, Ph.D:

There are many reports in the literature of Type-I diabetes emerging after mumps vaccination. In 1997, Sinaiotis and colleagues reported the onset of Type-I diabetes one month after receipt of mumps vaccine in a 6.5 year old boy. In 1991, Pawlowski and Gries described an 11-year old boy who had mumps disease at age 16 months and then received measles-mumps vaccine 5 months prior to the emergence of Type-I diabetes; he had severe abdominal pain and fever one week after vaccination. In 1984, Otten and colleagues reported three cases of Type-I diabetes with onset in one case 10 days and, in other cases, 3 weeks after mumps vaccination in children 3,2 and 16 years of age. In 1986, Helmke and colleagues reported seven children who developed Type-I diabetes in the second to fourth week following mumps or measles-mumps vaccination.

Soy and Type 1 Diabetes in Children

Contrary to popular belief that soy is a healthy food, evidence reveals that soy consumption has been linked to numerous disorders, including infertility, increased cancer and infantile leukemia, **Type1 diabetes**, and precocious puberty in children have been fed soy formula. Soy oil is the most widely used oil in the U.S., accounting for more than 75 percent of our total vegetable fats and oil intake. And most of our **soy products are now genetically engineered**.

Type 1 diabetes is slightly more common in males than in females.

Could a Cold Virus Trigger TYPE I Diabetes ? Victor Marchione, MD wrote:

Type 1 diabetes is known as an autoimmune disease. This means that your own immune system attacks and destroys insulin-producing cells in the pancreas. Medical experts are not completely sure what causes the immune system to behave this way, but it could be triggered by something entirely unexpected: a cold-like virus.

Australian researchers recently conducted a review of a number of studies and found there was a strong association between entero -viruses and the development of type 1 diabetes. In fact, children with diabetes were 10 times more likely to have had an enterovirus infection than children without the disease! For the study, the research team analyzed 24 papers and two abstracts involving 4,448 individuals to see if there was an association between type 1 diabetes and enterovirus (a virus that lives in the gut) infection. The data showed an especially strong association among children.

Enteroviruses usually cause cold or flu symptoms, fever, muscle aches, rash or even meningitis, they noted. Recently, there has been a worldwide increase in the incidence of childhood type 1 diabetes, especially in children under five, which the researchers now think could be the result of more exposure to these viruses.

Type 2 diabetes: Type 2 diabetes has strong genetic links, meaning that type 2 diabetes tends to run in families. Several genes have been identified and more are under study which may relate to the causes of type 2 diabetes. Risk factors for developing type 2 diabetes include the following:

- -High blood pressure
- -High blood triglyceride (fat) levels
- -High Level of bad cholesterol
- -Thyroid disorder
- -**Helicobacter pylori** infection
- **The shocking link between inflammation and diabetes most doctors miss!!!**
- -Gestational diabetes or giving birth to a baby weighing more than 9 pounds

Chapter I

- -High-fat diet .

- -High alcohol and carbonated beverages intake

- -Sedentary   lazy   lifestyle ; which   includes sitting, reading, watching TV and computer use for much of the day with little or no walking or physical exercise.

- -Stress and diabetes are common partners.

- -Obesity or being overweight .

- -Smoking which causes blood venous insufficiency.

- -Lack of sleep is linked to both diabetes and high blood pressure.

- - Pesticides represents a hidden risk which causes diabetes. This is a shocking warning by the National Institutes of Health

- -Ethnicity, particularly when a close relative had type 2 diabetes or gestational diabetes: certain groups, such as African Americans, Native Americans, Hispanic Americans, and Japanese Americans, have a greater risk of developing type 2 diabetes than non-Hispanic whites.

- -Aging: Increasing age is a significant risk factor for type 2 diabetes. Risk begins to rise significantly at about age 45 years, and rises considerably after age 65 years.

- **Could Wheat Allergy Play a Role in Diabetes Development?**

- An abnormal response to **wheat Gluten proteins** may tip a person's delicately poised immune system into developing type-1 diabetes, suggests a study from Canada.

Writing in the journal Diabetes, researchers from the Ottawa Hospital Research Institute and the University of Ottawa report that almost half of the 42 type-1 diabetics tested in their study had an abnormal immune response to wheat proteins.

"The presence of an [immune response] to [wheat proteins] in a subset of patients indicates a diabetes-related inflammatory state in the gut immune tissues associated with defective oral tolerance and possibly gut barrier dysfunction," wrote the researchers, led by Dr. Fraser Scott.

11

Type-1 diabetes occurs when people are not able to produce any insulin after the cells in the pancreas have been damaged, thought to be an autoimmune response. The immune system is thought to mistakenly attack the pancreas, the organ that regulates blood sugar. The disease is most common among people of European descent, with around two million Europeans and North Americans affected.

In addition, the incidence of the disease is on the rise at about three per cent per year, according to a study published last year in the *Archives of Disease in Childhood*. The number of new cases is estimated to rise 40 per cent between 2000 and 2010.

"The immune system has to find the perfect balance to defend the body against foreign invaders without hurting itself or over-reacting to the environment and this can be particularly challenging in the gut, where there is an abundance of food and bacteria," said Dr Scott.

"Our research suggests that people with certain genes may be more likely to develop an over-reaction to wheat and possibly other foods in the gut and this may tip the balance with the immune system and make the body more likely to develop other immune problems, such as type-1 diabetes."

With a growing number of people suffering from coeliac disease, the food industry is already producing more wheat-free foods, adding to the burgeoning 'free-from' market, which has been enjoying sales growth of over 300 per cent in the UK since 2000, according to market analyst Mintel.

THIAMINE LACK CAUSES DIABETES

Diabetes is associated with nerve damage, eye problems and kidney damage. Extended periods of high blood sugar causes your body to lose essential nutrients that it needs. One of those essential nutrients was discovered by a breaking study done in 2003 from the University of Essex, scientists realized that diabetics suffer from extreme deficiencies of thiamine.

The importance of thiamine as an essential diabetes fighting ingredient has become very clear over the past few years. Some

Chapter I

researchers have reason to believe that the key to fighting all of those diabetic complications might be as simple as a single vitamin: vitamin B1, otherwise known as thiamine.

Thiamine has always been one of my own personal favorites. Most doctors choose not to educate themselves about this great nutrient, which is very safe, non-allergenic and incredibly effective treatment - especially for diabetes.

Thiamine is needed for carbohydrate metabolism and for the release of energy from food. It also aids the heart and the nervous system to function well.

Other Functions of Thiamine :

Prevents the inflammation of nerves.

Promotes regeneration of damaged tissue

Prevents oxidation and neutralizes free radicals

It is anti-stress,and strengthens the immune system.

Here are some symptoms you may be suffering from if you are lacking Thiamine.

Depression, anxiety, fatigue, insomnia, headaches, indigestion, diarrhea, constipation, poor appetite, weight loss, numbness or burning sensation in the hands and feet, intolerance to pain, sensitivity to noises, edema, low blood pressure, anemia, low metabolism, shortness of breathe, heart palpitation, heart failure and enlarged heart on x-ray.

You can see now how important Thiamine is for everyone on a daily basis

Can Bread Cause Diabetes?

We know that food -- specifically too much of it and the resulting weight gain -- causes type 2 diabetes. But could what we eat be a cause of type 1 diabetes? Perhaps, says a new study that has linked wheat consumption to development of type 1 diabetes in young people (generally age 40 and younger), in a finding that has surprised many doctors and scientists. This is research that Daily Health News contributing editor, Andrew L. Rubman, ND, says is "quite amazing and hugely important."

Unlike the more common type 2, type 1 diabetes is a progressive autoimmune disorder that people develop early in life. Some cases have clear genetic roots, but scientists have believed that environmental factors could also play a role -- including, possibly, something in the diet. This small study from the University of Ottawa demonstrates that one factor may be wheat consumption.

Wheat and Diabetes Link

The study included 42 men and women, mostly young adults, with type 1 diabetes and a control group of 22 similar young people who did not have diabetes or any other known autoimmune disease. Researchers wanted to see how the immune systems in those with diabetes would respond to wheat.What they learned:Twenty of the 42 diabetes patients were "high responders" to wheat, which was demonstrated by heightened immune system activity. According to the researchers, this response was found at a "significantly higher" rate than in the control group. Also, nearly all patients in this group carried a gene known to increase risk of diabetes.

Wheat and What Else?

Wheat cannot be said to actually have caused the onset of diabetes in these patients, Dr. Rubman said, but the study does make a case that wheat consumption (specifically gluten found in wheat, rye and barley) could play a role in turning the genetic diabetes switch to "on" for those who carry the risk gene. Other factors may be involved too, he noted, while affirming that this study provides an early seed of knowledge that may someday help people avoid diabetes onset, or at the very least reduce the distress it causes. While there is more to learn, it is a healthy habit for all, especially children, to limit wheat consumption, rotating it with assorted other grains in order to minimize its impact on the body.

Dr.Rubman says that gluten avoidance might prove useful for people who already have type 1 diabetes because it may reduce the impact of the disease. If you have this type of diabetes, try a gluten-free diet for four to six months to see if symptom severity and blood sugar control improve. If the answer is yes, Dr. Rubman advises staying gluten-free for life.

Source(s): Andrew L. Rubman, ND, Medical Director, Southbury Clinic for Traditional Medicines, Southbury, Connecticut. www.SouthburyClinic.com.

The Mercury and Diabetes Connection

Although many researchers disagree on the conclusions, holistic health practitioners have long thought that thimerosal, an organic mercury compound, used as a preservative in childhood vaccines could be a contributing factor to developing type 1 diabetes in children and adolescents as well as other diseases like autism.

Interestingly, however, before even receiving vaccines, over 300,000 U.S. infants are born already having been exposed to organic methylmercury in utero from their mothers through diet or environmental exposure! After birth, an infant can be additionally exposed to methylmercury through their mother's breast milk where it's stored! Could environmental mercury exposure, be contributing to the current diabetic epidemic?

It's highly possible, given the results of several recent studies which showed that inorganic mercury exposure caused either insulin receptor beta cell death, or dysfunction — where they secreted too little insulin resulting in elevated glucose levels.

One study showed that exposure to organic mercury (methylmercury) in fish, consumed in amounts under the EPA's current recommended fish/mercury levels actually caused beta cell dysfunction. Another study done on mice had the same findings with an additional result showing the insulin receptors and glucose levels returned to normal when the mercury exposure stopped.

What these studies suggest is we have to be a little more vigilant in the levels of mercury we are exposed to in order to help prevent the onset of diabetes.

CHAPTER II
TYPE 3 DIABETES

Mike Adam wrote (Source: Adams, Mike (June 10, 2010). "New Research: Electropollution can cause diabetes (type-3)." NaturalNews.com):

(Most people are familiar with type-1 diabetes and type-2 diabetes, but researchers have discovered a third type of diabetes; Type-3 diabetes, as they are calling it, affects people who are extra sensitive to electrical devices that emit "harmful" electricity.

Type-3 diabetics actually experience spikes in blood sugar and an increased heart rate when exposed to electrical pollution ("electropollution") from things like computers, televisions, cordless and mobile phones, and even compact fluorescent light bulbs.

Dr. Magda Havas, a PhD from Trent University in Canada, recently published the results of a study she conducted on the relationship between electromagnetic fields and diabetes in *Electromagnetic Biology and Medicine*. She explains how she and her team came to discover this about why electropollution is so dangerous for many people.

Blood sugar goes haywire

One of the most interesting finding in her study was that electro-sensitive people whose blood sugar decreases when they go for a walk outdoors actually experience **an increase in blood sugar** when walking on a treadmill.

Treadmills, you see, are electrical devices that emit electrical pollution. But interestingly, even the physical exertion of walking on the treadmill did not make up for the blood sugar spiking effect of the EMFs emitted by the treadmills. Despite the exercise, in other words, type-3 diabetics experienced significant spikes in blood sugar when walking on the treadmill.

Dirty electricity is bad for everyone, but it is especially bad for people who are type-3 diabetics. And Dr. Havas explains in her study that even having an electrical device plugged into the wall near someone who is type-3 diabetic can cause them problems.

We have to rethink environmental influences of modern living

I find this research fascinating, not only because it proves that electromagnetic waves impact blood sugar and heart rate, but because there could be thousands, if not millions, of diabetics who may be suffering from a diabetes misdiagnosis right now. The reason I'm bringing this up is because a 54 year-old pre-diabetic man who participated in the study was found to experience serious blood sugar spikes **only when he was working in an urban environment around power lines or on his computer.** When he was out camping away from the city, his blood sugar was just fine.

The man tested his blood sugar every morning in different situations and his levels were always higher when electrical fields were nearby. On one of the mornings, he forgot to test himself prior to beginning work on the computer. His blood sugar levels were higher than normal, registering around 205 milligrams per deciliter (mg/dL). But after stepping away from the computer for only ten minutes, his levels dropped nearly 20 mg/dL. The degree to which electromagnetic pollution affects the body is clearly quite astonishing, and this study illustrates that. But it makes you wonder how many people have diabetes simply *because* of EMF pollution (and not solely due to their diet or lack of exercise, as we have been taught).

High EMFs gave this woman diabetes

Take the case of the 80 year-old woman whose house tested high for EMF pollution. Prior to installing a system of filters around her house designed to reduce "electro-smog" levels, her blood sugar was high and she was using insulin each day in order to balance her blood sugar levels. After installing the filters (which reduced EMF pollution by roughly 98 percent), the woman's blood sugar levels dropped by 33 percent and her insulin requirements plunged a whopping 75 percent!

This idea that reducing the electropollution of your house could drastically reduce a patient's need for insulin has never even registered in conventional (mainstream) medicine. Yet it could be a crucial understanding for tens of millions of diabetics around the world.

The study mentioned here classifies the type of diabetes caused by electromagnetic pollution as **type-3 diabetes**. While those with type-1 or type-2 diabetes can also have type-3, the data seems to indicate that a

18

Chapter II

person can also exclusively have type-3 without any overlay of the other two types. In other words, their diabetes may be *solely* due to electromagnetic pollution.

And since pre-diabetics can be pushed over the edge by EMF pollution, there is no telling how many people actually have type-3 rather than type-2 diabetes.

If you ask most mainstream medical "professionals", they will deny that type-3 diabetes even exists. According to most of them, the idea that electromagnetic pollution contributes to disease is some sort of whacked out conspiracy theory. But there's more to the study that you need to know...

Wireless signals interfere with the heart

For one portion of the study, Dr. Havas had patients lie down on a bed with a cordless phone placed two feet away from their heads. The phone was plugged into the wall, but for each testing session, the electricity was either on or off.

Neither the patient nor the doctor administering the test was aware of whether or not the phone was live or dead during each session. (This is what is known as a double-blind study, the type most respected in clinical trials).

At the completion of that part of the study, researchers observed that **EMF-sensitive patients experienced significant increases in their heart rates** during the sessions when the phone was being powered and emitting radio signals. When it was turned off, these same patients returned back to their normal heart rates *almost instantaneously*.

Why is this important? First of all, a double-blind study is the litmus test used in the medical profession to verify that a study is legitimate. Since nobody involved knew when the power was on or off, the results are completely unbiased and hold a lot more effect than if it had been conducted a different way.

Secondly, it illustrates that EMF pollution really *does* speed up the heart rates of certain people. And since a rapid pulse is one of the many symptoms of diabetes, it seems reasonable to suspect that EMF pollution could be a *fundamental cause* of diabetic symptoms for a significant

19

portion of the diabetic population.

This makes you wonder about the harm caused by mammograms, CT scans and other medical scanning technologies that blast the body with electromagnetic radiation.

Electromagnetic radiation leads to many diseases, including cancer

Our bodies are constantly barraged by electromagnetic radiation from numerous electronic sources, and most people don't think twice about this high level of exposure (probably because many don't even realize it's there), but the truth is that all this EMF pollution is leading to widespread illness.

Most of the recent research on EMF pollution has focused on cell phones, which makes sense because people take their cell phones with them everywhere they go and when they use them, they often hold them right next to their skulls. Cell phone radiation is probably one of the most dangerous EMF polluters because the devices remain in very close contact with the body for long periods of time.

A 2008 study published in *New Scientist* revealed that cell phone radiation causes human cell proteins to improperly express themselves. Similar studies also found that the radiation damages living DNA, creates leakages in the blood-brain barrier, and increases estrogen and adrenaline levels, disrupting hormone balance.

According to one statistic from a 2008 study, adults who use a cell phone over the course of a decade increase their chances of developing brain cancer by **40 percent**. Even worse, a Swedish study found that people who start using a cell phone before the age of 20 increase their risk of developing a brain tumor by 500 percent!!

Mainstream science holds conflicting views (as usual).

Of course, many in the medical establishment simply deny that electro-smog has anything to do with health or disease. And it doesn't matter how many studies are conducted on the matter; *many continue to insist that there is not enough evidence that EMFs cause any harm.*

Not everyone feels this way, of course, but sadly most of today's experts seem unable (or unwilling) to put two and two together and make the connection between electromagnetic pollution and disease.

Chapter II

There are many contributors to disease in our environment. EMFs represent just one. But to deny that electromagnetic pollution is harmful is quite narrow minded. Dr. Havas' study provides more than enough evidence that at least *some* people are suffering because of the electrical devices that surround them.

Our world, of course, is full of electromagnetic devices -- and some of them may surprise you. A typical hair dryer, for example, emits an explosion of electromagnetic radiation that's usually aimed right at the skull. Typical office environments shower employees with electropollution from fluorescent lighting, and even exercise gyms can subject visitors to a dense field of electromagnetic pollution (from all the electronic exercise machines).

It all gives credence to the idea of getting into nature more often, doesn't it? If you're sensitive to electropollution, the farther away you get from the city, the better you'll feel. No wonder most people innately gravitate to such natural environments like forests, lakes and ocean beaches.

So, does all this research mean we should all get rid of our phones and computers and return to the pre-information age? You could always join an Amish community. They're remarkably healthy, and part of that may be due to their lack of electropollution.

But for mainstream people, a more practical solution is to install some EMF filters around your home.

Some solutions for electromagnetic pollution.

As mentioned in the study, *home EMF filters* are one of the best ways to reduce or eliminate the stray electrical signals that plague your house. These filters will capture electrical "noise" from things like televisions, computers and phones, and return it back into the line or into the ground. These can be connected to the outlets where these devices are plugged in.

Keeping Wi-Fi devices like cell phones and wireless routers *away from your body* as much as possible is another good idea. If you have a wireless router at home, place it away from areas where people sleep or spend a lot of time. Even having it just a few feet farther away can make a big difference in a reduction of the electropollution exposure from it.

When charging your cell phone, plug it in across the room from you. Especially at night when you are sleeping, it is best to turn off as many electrical devices as possible and to keep them away from your bed when sleeping. And beware of electric blankets: They produce a very strong electromagnetic field.

Try to use the speakerphone as much as possible when talking on the phone, or use an "air-tube" device that stops the signal short before it reaches your head. *Never* walk around with an idle bluetooth attached to your head, because these devices deliver a steady stream of EMF radiation directly into your head. I would recommend not using one at all, but if you do use one, take it off when not in use.

It's also a good idea to keep your phone in your pocket or purse *only when necessary*, and to keep it away from your body at all other times. Cell phones are intermittently communicating with network towers, so the closer they are to our bodies, the more radiation we are exposed to. So if you're not going to be using it for a while, *just turn it off*.

Finally, it is crucial to *maintain a healthy diet* and *get plenty of outdoor exercise*. Eating lots of nutrient-rich foods, drinking plenty of clean water, and minimizing intake of toxic preservatives, food additives, and refined sugars will do wonders to build a strong and vibrant neurological system that will resist some of the impact of electromagnetic pollution.

The reason I mention *outdoor* exercise is because, just like in the study, certain indoor exercise equipment like treadmills can actually cause more harm than good (for certain people). So go outside and take a walk or a jog. The sunshine will boost your vitamin D levels and the fresh air will help rejuvenate your system. (Just be sure to stay away from the power lines.)

Increased risk of Alzheimer's

The new diabetes type also strengthens scientists' belief that people with diabetes have an increased risk of suffering from Alzheimer's disease (by up to 65%).

Chapter II

Researchers at the medical school discovered that many type 2 diabetics have deposits of a protein in their pancreas which is similar to the protein deposits found in the brain tissue of Alzheimer's sufferers.

Dr Suzanne de la Monte, who led the research, and her colleagues studied rodents and post-mortem brain tissue from people with Alzheimer's and found that insulin and its related proteins are actually produced in the brain, and that reduced levels of both are linked to Alzheimer's disease.

Discovery that insulin is produced in the brain and it's decrease raises possibility of Type 3 diabetes linked to Alzheimer's Disease and changes the way we view the disease.

Researchers at Rhode Island Hospital and Brown Medical School have discovered that insulin and its related proteins are produced in the brain, and that reduced levels of both are linked to Alzheimer's disease.

"What we found is that insulin is not just produced in the pancreas, but also in the brain. And we discovered that insulin and its growth factors, which are necessary for the survival of brain cells, contribute to the progression of Alzheimer's," says senior author Suzanne M. de la Monte, a neuropathologist at Rhode Island Hospital and a professor of pathology at Brown Medical School. "This raises the possibility of a Type 3 diabetes."

It has previously been known that insulin resistance, a characteristic of diabetes, is tied to neurodegeneration. While scientists have suspected a link between diabetes and Alzheimer's disease, this is the first study to provide evidence of that connection.

By studying a gene abnormality in rats that blocks insulin signaling in the brain, researchers found that insulin and IGF I and II are all expressed in neurons in several regions in the brain.

Additionally, researchers determined that a drop in insulin production in the brain contributes to the degeneration of brain cells, an early symptom of Alzheimer's. "These abnormalities do not correspond to Type 1 or Type 2 diabetes, but reflect a different and more complex disease process that originates in the CNS (central nervous system)," the paper states.

23

Dr. Mansour

By looking at postmortem brain tissue from people diagnosed with Alzheimer's disease, researchers discovered that growth factors are not produced at normal levels in the hippocampus - the part of the brain responsible for memory. The absence of these growth factors, in turn, causes cells in other parts of the brain to die. Reserachers found that insulin and IGF I were significantly reduced in the frontal cortex, hippocampus and hypothalamus - all areas that are affected by the progression of Alzheimer's. Conversely, in the cerebellum, which is generally not affected by Alzheimer's, scientists did not see the same drop in insulin and I GF I.

"Now that scientists have pinpointed insulin and its growth factors as contributors to Alzheimer's, this opens the way for targeted treatment to the brain and changes the way we view Alzheimer's disease," de la Monte says.

The study was supported by grants from the National Institute of Alcoholism and Alcohol Abuse and from a COBRE award from the National Institutes of Health.

These findings are reported in the March issue of the Journal of Alzheimer's Disease (http://www.j-alz.com),

CHAPTER III

DIABETES COMPLICATIONS

Complications Are What Is Killing Diabetics

Diabetics aren't dying because they don't know how to lower glucose — they're dying from complications .Chemical drugs have failed to protect diabetics against deadly complications!!

Glucose-lowering drugs are rarely effective in the long term and do absolutely nothing to reverse the causes of diabetes: insulin resistance in diabetics cells.

In truth, **no glucose-lowering drug has ever been shown to produce a reliable reduction in diabetic complications.** Neither has aggressive glucose monitoring. Moreover diabetes drugs have very dangerous side effects on liver, kidney ,heart,sex ,eyes,.. etc.

You Can control glucose" and Die from Diabetes! :

A shocking study in 2008 proved it...

A group of Type 2 patients were told to aggressively maintain their blood sugar levels at 6.0% or lower with medications. After four years, these patients suffered significantly more heart attacks and a higher rate of death compared to patients whose levels were between 7.0 and 7.9%.

In short, they were following their doctor's orders to a "T." But the results were so dismaying that the study had to be canceled early to protect the remaining patients. The medical community was stunned. No one had ever questioned the safety of driving down glucose levels like this. It was always "assumed" to be the right thing to do.

Glucose Monitoring Won't Save Your Life

Another shocker: Vigilant glucose monitoring does nothing to prevent diabetic complications and this is proven conclusively by two studies published in the British Medical Journal.

The first study split a group of newly-diagnosed Type 2 patients into equal self-monitoring and no-monitoring groups. After 12 months, the diabetes (as measured by A1C testing) was no better in the self-monitoring group.

The second study divided a separate population of Type 2 patients into three groups: No monitoring, moderate monitoring, and intense monitoring. Not only did SMBG (Self-Monitoring Of Blood Glucose)fail to improve diabetes control, it also cost more. More importantly, monitoring actually decreased the patients' quality of life.

Despite this well-published research, most doctors continue to recommend aggresive glucose self-monitoring. One has to wonder if the cost of test strips and glucose monitors has anything to do with this.

The International Diabetes Federation (IDF) listed a number of short and long-term diabetes complications as follows:

Short-Term Complications:

- ### Low Bblood Sugar (Hypoglycemia)

A person who takes insulin is going to face the problem of their blood sugar falling too low at some point which is called **hypoglycemia** . Hypoglycemia can be corrected rapidly by eating some sugar. If it is not corrected it can lead to the person losing consciousness and falling into coma.

It is important that the person with diabetes recognizes the signs of hypoglycemia.

- ### Diabetic Ketoacidosis(DKA)

When the body breaks down fats, acidic waste products called ketones are produced. The body cannot tolerate large amounts of ketones and will try to get rid of them through the urine. However, the body cannot release all the ketones and they build up in your blood, causing ketoacidosis. Ketoacidosis is a severe condition caused by lack of insulin. It mainly affects people with type 1 diabetes. In extreme cases ketoacidosis can be fatal. Prolonged alcoholism may lead to alcoholic ketoacidosis. Fasting leads to ketosis but not ketoacidosis. Ketoacidosis can be smelled on a person's breath. This is due to acetone, a direct byproduct of the spontaneous decomposition of aceto-acetic acid. It is often described as smelling like fruit or nail polish remover.

- ### Lactic Aacidosis

Lactic acidosis is the build up of lactic acid in the body. Cells make lactic acid when they use glucose for energy. The condition typically occurs when cells receive too little oxygen and it is characterized by low pH in body tissues. If too much lactic acid stays in the body, the balance tips and the person begins to feel ill. Lactic acidosis is rare and mainly

Chapter III ──────────────

affects people with type 2 diabetes.Some diabetes drugs such as Metformin cause lactic acidosis.

- **Bacterial/Fungal Infections**

People with diabetes are more prone to bacterial and fungal infections. Bacterial infections include sties and boils. Fungal infections include athlete's foot, ringworm and vaginal infections.

Long-Term Complications:

Most long-term complications of diabetes result from venous insuffeciency and poor blood circulations to brain,heart,kidney ,penis and foot.Some diabetes drugs such as Metformin cause venous insuffeciency the thing which complicates the diabetics health condition.

- **Eye Disease (Retinopathy)**

Eye disease, or retinopathy, is the **leading cause of blindness** and visual impairment in adults in developed societies. About 2% of all people who have had diabetes for 15 years become blind, while about 10% develop a severe visual impairment.

- **Kidney Disease (Nephropathy)**

Diabetes is the leading cause of kidney disease
(nephropathy). About one third of all people with diabetes develop kidney disease and approximately 20% of people with type 1 diabetes develop kidney (renal)failure.

- **Nerve Disease (Neuropathy)**

Diabetic nerve disease, or neuropathy affects at least half of all people with diabetes. There are different types of nerve disease which can result in a loss of sensation in the feet or in some cases the hands, pain in the foot and problems with the functioning of different parts of the body including the heart, the eye, the stomach, the bladder and the penis. A lack of sensation in the feet can lead to people with diabetes injuring their feet without realizing it. These injuries can lead to ulcers and possibly amputation.

- ## Diseases of the Circulatory System:

- ### Heart Attack

Disease of the circulatory system, or cardiovascular disease, accounts for 75% of all deaths among people with diabetes of European origin. In the USA, coronary heart disease is present in between 8% and 20% of people with diabetes over 45 years of age. Their risk of heart disease is 2-4 times higher than those who do not have diabetes. It is the main cause of disability and death for people with type 2 diabetes.

Scientists have found that garlic has "significant" potential for preventing "cardiomyopathy." This type of heart disease a leading cause of death in people with diabetes, making it a very significant health issue. The new study, which also explains why diabetics are at high risk for cardiomyopathy, appears in the Journal of Agricultural and Food Chemistry. The group of researchers had hints from past studies that garlic might protect against heart disease. And that garlic might help control the abnormally high blood sugar levels that occur in diabetes. But they realized that few studies had been done specifically on garlic's effects on "diabetic cardiomyopathy".

- ### Stroke and Diabetes

If you have diabetes, it's important to understand your increased risk of stroke. Multiple studies have shown that people with diabetes are at greater risk for stroke compared to people without diabetes regardless of the number of health risk factors they have. Overall, the health risk of cardiovascular disease (including stroke) is two-and-a-half times higher in men and women with diabetes compared to people without diabetes.

- ### High Blood Pressure(Hypertension) and Diabetes

Having diabetes increases your risk of developing high blood pressure and other cardiovascular problems, because diabetes adversely affects the arteries, predisposing them to atherosclerosis (hardening of the arteries). Atherosclerosis can cause high blood pressure, which if not treated, can lead to blood vessel damage, stroke, heart failure, heart attack, or kidney failure.

- ### Foot Gangrene and Amputation

Diabetic Gangrene is a condition that involves the death and decay of tissue, usually in the extremities. Diabetic Gangrene leads after a while

Chapter III ─────────

to fingers and foot amputation. People with diabetes are 15 to 40 times more likely to require lower-limb amputation compared to the general population. The major causes of diabetic gangrene is poor blood circulation and the disability of blood to reach foot in a sufficient manner. Cardiovascular problems, and smoking are added to the most common causes.

- **Diabetes and Erectile Dysfunction(Impotence)**

Studies Show Diabetes is linked to loss of libido and Erectile Dysfunction.

Middle aged and older adults are interested in sexual activity, but diabetes impairs libido and can result in erectile dysfunction, a new study shows:

Researchers in Chicago say men diagnosed with diabetes are more likely to express a lack of interest in sex, but also to experience erectile dysfunction.

Scientists at the University of Chicago Medical Center conducted a study of nearly 2,000 people between the ages of 57 and 85.

The study found that about 70% of men and 62% of women with diabetes and sexual partners were found to engage in sexual activity two or three times a month comparable to people without diabetes.

The study also found that:

- Men were more likely to express a lack of interest in sex if they had diabetes.

- Men also were more likely to suffer erectile dysfunction if they had diabetes.

- Women as well as men with diabetes reported a higher rate of orgasm difficulty, including climaxing too quickly for men, or not at all, which was reported by both men and women.

- Only 19% of women compared to 47% of men, all with diabetes, had discussed sexual problems with a doctor, and men were more likely to talk about it than women.

- Men in the study regardless of age or diabetes status were more likely than women to be married or living with a partner, and more men than women said they were sexually active.

- ## Link between Insulin and Cholesterol

Researchers are still figuring out exactly how diabetes changes cholesterol levels at the microscopic cellular level. They do know that high levels of insulin in the blood tend to adversely affect the number of cholesterol particles in the blood. High insulin levels act to raise the amount of LDL cholesterol (the "bad cholesterol") that tends to form plaques in arteries, and lower the number of HDL cholesterol particles ("good cholesterol") that help to clear out dangerous plaques before they break off to cause a heart attack or stroke. Diabetes also tends to cause higher levels of triglycerides, another type of fat circulating in the blood.

Similarly, high cholesterol can also be a predictor of diabetes; elevated cholesterol levels are often seen in people with insulin resistance, even before they have developed full-blown diabetes. When LDL levels start to climb, experts recommend paying close attention to blood sugar control and starting a diet and exercise regimen to help stave off diabetes and cardiovascular disease. This is especially important if you have a family history of heart disease.

- ## Diabetes and Memory Loss

There is a shocking link between too much sugar and memory loss!

Though this fact is not mentioned in the medical books of diabetes it is expected since diabetes causes poor blood circulation throughout the whole body and this affects blood transport to eyes,heart, kidney,penis,foot as well as brain!!!

Links Between Diabetes and Cancer

Serena Gordon A HealthDay Reporter wrote:

WEDNESDAY, June 16 (HealthDay News) - People with diabetes may have something else to be concerned about an increased risk of cancer, according to a new consensus report produced by experts recruited jointly by the American Cancer Society and the American Diabetes Association.

Diabetes, primarily type 2 diabetes, has been linked to certain cancers, though experts aren't sure if the disease itself leads to the increased risk or if shared risk factors, such as obesity, may be to blame.

Other research has suggested that some diabetes treatments, such as certain insulins, may also be associated with the development of some

Chapter III ──────────────────

cancers. But the evidence isn't conclusive, and it's difficult to tease out whether the insulin is responsible for the association or other risk factors associated with diabetes could be the root of the link. For more information about the dangers of insulin you can read the book: **Insulin: Our silent killer by Thomas Smith.**

As for the possible insulin-and-cancer link, Harlan said that because a weak association was found, it's definitely an area that needs to be pursued further. But, he said, that doesn't mean that anyone should change the way they're managing their diabetes.

The consensus report is published in the July/August issue of: *Cancer Journal for Clinicians.*

The experts found evidence of an association between diabetes and an increased risk of liver, pancreas, endometrial, colon/rectal, breast and bladder cancer. Interestingly, they found evidence that diabetes is associated with a reduced risk of prostate cancer.

"There's a strong consensus that there is a link between diabetes and cancer, and there are some very plausible biologic links," said the report's lead author, Dr. Edward Giovannucci, a professor of nutrition and epidemiology at the Harvard School of Public Health in Boston. He said that insulin, and insulin-like growth factors, can promote some cancers, and that many people with type 2 diabetes have high levels of circulating insulin, sometimes for years before they're diagnosed with diabetes.

And, he said, there's definitely an overlap in some of the risk factors for both type 2 diabetes and cancer, especially obesity.

The panel also found research that suggests the commonly used type 2 diabetes medication, metformin, might offer users some protection against cancer. Giovannucci said this may be because the drug reduces insulin resistance and lowers the need for additional insulin, or that metformin may act on cells in other direct or indirect ways.

Giovannucci said that the most important message to take away from this research is the "profound effects that lifestyle changes can have on your risk of diabetes and your risk of cancer."

He said it's not always the most popular message, but to lower the risk of cancer, it's important to reduce your body weight, exercise, improve your diet and avoid smoking.

Alice Bender, the nutrition communications manager for the American Institute for Cancer Research (AICR), said she wasn't surprised by the findings in the consensus report. "What we're seeing is that there are a lot of commonalities between chronic diseases and their risk factors," she said.

Bender agreed with Giovannucci's suggestions and said the AICR recommends three guidelines for everyone: Maintain a healthy body weight; be physically active for at least 30 minutes a day; and, eat a mostly plant-based diet that's healthy and varied.

Bender also emphasized the need to moderate the consumption of alcohol, which means no more than one drink per day for women and no more than two drinks per day for men.

Type II Diabetes & Alzheimer

Insulin resistant people with type 2 diabetes are more likely to develop plaques in their brains which are associated with Alzheimer's disease.

A study looked at 135 elderly participants who were monitored for signs of Alzheimer's disease for 10 to 15 years. After they died, researchers conducted autopsies on their brains and that those who had high blood sugar levels while they were alive also tended to have the plaques.

According to Reuters: "Twenty-one participants, or 16 percent, developed Alzheimer's disease before they died and plaques were found in all of their brains. But the autopsies also found plaques in other participants who had abnormally high blood sugar levels.

Plaques were found in 72 percent of people with insulin resistance and 62 percent of those with no indication of insulin resistance, the researchers wrote.

"The point is that insulin resistance may possibly accelerate plaque pathology (development)," Sasaki wrote."

This is not the first time researchers have connected diabetes with Alzheimer's. In fact, Alzheimer's disease was tentatively dubbed "type 3

Chapter III ——————————————

diabetes" in early 2005 when researchers realized that your pancreas is not the only organ that produces insulin.

Your brain also produces insulin, and this brain insulin is necessary for the survival of your brain cells. But interestingly, while low insulin levels in your body are associated with improved health, the opposite appears to be true when it comes to your brain insulin.

A drop in insulin production in your brain contributes to the degeneration of brain cells, and studies have found that people with lower levels of insulin and insulin receptors in their brain often have Alzheimer's disease.

A 2004 study also revealed that people with diabetes have a 65 percent higher risk of developing Alzheimer's disease.

New Evidence Strengthening the Link Between Diabetes and Alzheimer's Disease

According to this recent Japanese study, insulin resistance and/or diabetes appear to accelerate the development of plaque in your brain, which is a hallmark of Alzheimer's.

This study, which had a very long observation period, further strengthens the link between these two diseases, as different as they may otherwise appear to be.

In this study, which monitored 135 people for 10 to 15 years, 16 percent developed Alzheimer's disease before they died, and autopsy showed they all had plaque in their brains.

CHAPTER IV

DIABETES DRUGS : EFFECTS & SIDE EFFECTS

The Diabetes Industry

Thomas Smith wrote:Today's diabetes industry is a massive community that has grown step by step from its dubious origins in the early 20th century. In the last 80 years it has become enormously successful at shutting out competitive voices that attempt to point out the fraud involved in modern diabetes treatment. It has matured into a religion. And, like all religions, it depends heavily upon the faith of the believer. So successful has it become that it verges on blasphemy to suggest that, in most cases, the kindly high priest with the stethoscope draped prominently around his neck is a charlatan and a fraud. In the large majority of cases, he has never cured a single case of diabetes in his entire medical career.

The financial and political influence of this medical community has almost totally subverted the original intent of our regulatory agencies. They routinely approve death-dealing, ineffective drugs with insufficient testing. Former commissioner of the FDA, Dr Herbert Ley, in testimony before a US Senate hearing, commented: "People think the FDA is protecting them. It isn't. What the FDA is doing and what the public thinks it's doing are as different as night and day.)

Why lowering blood sugar may be a mistake...?

by Buck Rizvi on July 8, 2010:

What most of us have been lead to believe is just not true.

Conventional medicine would have you believe that lowering your blood sugar is the be-all, end-all solution to type 2 diabetes.

But what if that is a mistake that misses the REAL underlying trigger of not just what causes type 2 diabetes, but all major age-related illnesses?

You see, elevated blood sugar is just a SYMPTOM of underlying metabolic, physiologic, and biochemical processes that are out of balance.

Lowering blood sugar with medications does NOT address the underlying triggers that give rise to the high blood sugar in the first place.

This may surprise you, but many of the methods used to lower blood sugar such as insulin or oral hypoglycemic drugs actually make the problem WORSE!!

This happens because these methods actually increase the levels of another substance in your body that is the true trigger of the misery that over 125 million Americans suffer from.

This substance is the single most important trigger that leads to rapid and premature aging and all its resultant diseases, including heart disease, stroke, dementia, and cancer.

But when you shift your focus from trying to manage blood sugar, as millions unfortunately incorrectly do now, to fixing the underlying problems that cause excessive levels of this particularly deadly trigger, remarkable things can occur, such as:

- Weight loss, particularly around the belly...
- Improved energy...
- Better mental clarity...
- More stable, enjoyable mood...
- Better memory...
- Reduced joint pain...
- Improvement in blood sugar and hemoglobin A1c...
- Lower blood pressure and cholesterol...

How to Reverse Your Diabetes without Medications

Read Chapters – 19,24 and 25 of this book.

Drug companies make billions of dollars every year "managing" diabetes and other debilitating conditions with their expensive drugs. These chronic diseases are their bread-and-butter—so they're doing everything in their power to hush up this inexpensive breakthrough and sweep it under the rug.

And they'll stop at nothing to keep the truth away from you.

Chapter IV

There is no reason in the world why you should EVER suffer a debilitating disease like diabetes when an effective treatment like natural herbs can make it disappear. None!

And there's no reason you should go broke fending off age-related conditions that can make your life miserable, just so drug companies can "make their numbers" and impress Wall Street.

Now, though, you can actually do something about it. This amazing health-restoring therapy that helps halt diabetes is detailed in Chapters 19, 24 and 25.

Having diabetes is no big deal these days. By monitoring your blood sugar and following your doctor's orders, you can enjoy a normal life and escape diabetic complications, including nerve damage, going blind and losing limbs through amputation -- not to mention heart attack, stroke and Alzheimer's disease.

Why glucose monitoring is a waste of time and money for people with Type 2.

Recent studies proving that current diabetes drugs (and insulin injections!) provide zero protection against its horrible complications.

Why doctors are ignoring the most successful natural diabetes treatment in the world -- even though it's been thoroughly proven to reverse diabetes.

Diabetes Death Pills

If you are concerned about your blood sugar, did you realize that most diabetes drugs fail to work for HALF of all patients?*

That's why the TV ads tell you to "Ask your doctor if this medication is right for you."

Yet the only way he can tell is by trying the drug on you first -- because each of us responds differently to the same treatment. That means...

Diabetes patients are guinea pigs in a massive experiment

And the chances that you'll get a good response to a given drug are NOT in your favor. Here's why...

To receive FDA approval, a drug only needs to prove that it's better than a sugar pill. So a drug that works 20% of the time gets approved for use -- even though it produces absolutely no improvement in 80% of patients.

That's bad enough, but the story gets worse...

Drug companies pressure the FDA to "fast-track" approval of new drugs to get them on the market sooner.

Here is a Summary of the Most Anti-Diabetic Chemical Drugs :

Orinase. In 1957, the Upjohn Company introduced this new blood sugar-lowering "wonder drug," promising it could halt diabetes and prevent its progression in symptomless patients (what we now refer to as prediabetes). It wasn't until 1970 that independent researchers concluded **Orinase actually was killing patients** -- causing more than twice the heart disease deaths compared to doing absolutely nothing.

Phenformin. Discovered in 1958 and marketed by Ciba-Geigy, **it was banned in 1977** due to a high risk of lactic acidosis, which proved fatal in 50% of cases.

Rezulin. The FDA fast-tracked its approval in January 1997 -- and numerous liver failure cases began to surface within months. A high-ranking FDA called Rezulin one of the most dangerous drugs in America, but it wasn't **banned until March 2000**, after being implicated in **391 deaths**. (During that time it earned more than $2 billion for its manufacturer, Warner-Lambert.)

Avandia. By 2007, there were 18 different glucose-lowering medications being prescribed, including one of the bestselling diabetes drug in history, Avandia from GlaxoSmithKline. The FDA fast-tracked it, too; even though none of these new drugs were even proven to be effective or safe -- especially when compared to simple diet and lifestyle modifications.

In fact, an earth-shaking study published in the New England Journal of Medicine showed just the opposite: **Avandia actually increased the risk of heart attack by 43%** -- and **cardiovascular deaths by a whopping 64%** -- compared to patients not on the drug. That meant that not taking Avandia doubled a Type 2 patient's chances of

Chapter IV

avoiding a cardiovascular event (the cause of death in 75% of diabetes patients).

Incredibly, Glaxo hid the drug's dangers from the public!

Senate investigations begun in early 2010 showed that as far back as 2003, Glaxo's own studies revealed that Avandia caused serious heart problems, but that the company hid this from the public and the FDA.

A report published in 2007 by Cleveland Clinic's Steven Nissen showed that it increased the risk of heart attacks in more than 40 percent of Avandia users. The FDA's drug safety expert, David Graham also revealed that Avandia was responsible for heart problems, which sometimes turned fatal, in 66,000 to 200,000 people.

Even though Avandia may have been responsible for as many as 800,000 deaths, Glaxo continued to aggressively market it (it's still on the market!), persuading doctors to recommend the drug .

Avandia was withdrawn from market - October 2010

GlaxoSmithKline's Avandia, once the world's best-selling diabetes drug, will be withdrawn from the market in Europe and sales will be limited in the United States because of an increased risk of heart attacks, regulators said in decisions announced almost simultaneously.

Avandia, has been withdrawn from New Zealand's market after "Medsafe Group Manager Dr Stewart Jessamine said a safety review had found New Zealand patients taking the drug suffered an increased risk of cardiovascular events," the New Zealand Herald reports.

An FDA panel recommended that Glaxo's anti diabetes drug, Avandia be either withdrawn from the market, or that the agency place restrictions on its use. It was a major blow to GlaxoSmithKline, but not entirely unexpexpected to Houston injury lawyers, given that Glaxo had come under such criticism from an FDA official last week.

Actos linked to heart risk and bladder cancer:

Dr. Allan Spreen wrote on 04/16/2011:

Many people consider Actos a safer alternative to other diabetes drugs, but it's not. Here's why...

It belongs to the same class of drugs as Avandia. As you'll recall, the FDA greatly restricts the use of Avandia because it may increase your heart attack risk. So, how about Actos? Could it increase heart attack risk too? Of course, it could. In fact, a 2010 study found that Actos caused **as many heart problems** as Avandia. Plus, the FDA is investigating a link between Actos and bladder cancer. I suspect they will find the longer you take Actos, the greater your risk.

A group of Italian researchers analyzed all the adverse events reported to the FDA between 2004 and 2009 for 15 diabetes drugs on the market, including Actos and metformin.

When they analyzed the reporting odds ratio (ROR), they found a "definite risk" linking Actos and bladder cancer. In fact, this week researchers published a report that found an association between Actos and a certain form of cancer. Plus, this isn't the first study to uncover a link between Actos and increased cancer risk

Glucophage. In the 1990s, a new class of sugar-lowering drugs made its appearance, including metformin, a drug similar to phenformin which debuted in 1994. Marketed under the brand name Glucophage, it's since become the best selling pill for Type 2 and prediabetes.

Metformin causes vitamin B12 deficiency

10/31/2010 - Long-term use of the popular diabetes drug metformin (originally marketed as Glucophage) may cause patients to develop a steadily worsening vitamin B12 deficiency, Dutch scientists have found.

"Our study shows that this decrease is not a transitory phenomenon, but persists and grows over time," wrote the Maastricht University Medical Center researchers in the *British Medical Journal.* "Metformin is considered a cornerstone in the treatment of diabetes and is the most frequently prescribed first line therapy for individuals with type 2 diabetes," the researchers wrote. "In addition, it is one of a few ... associated with improvements in cardiovascular morbidity and mortality, which is a major cause of death in patients with type 2 diabetes."

Earlier, short-term studies had found that use of the drug might lead to insufficient levels of the vitamin in the body. The new study confirmed this trend over the long term.

Chapter IV ────────────────────────────

"Metformin does ... induce vitamin B12 malabsorption, which may increase the risk of developing vitamin B12 deficiency -- a clinically important and treatable condition," the researchers wrote.

The researchers assigned 390 Type 2 diabetes patients at the outpatient clinics of three nonacademic hospitals to take either metformin or a placebo pill three times per day for more than four years. The average study participant had been diagnosed with diabetes 13 years prior and had been undergoing insulin treatment for seven years. Average participant age was 61.

Among those taking metformin, vitamin B12 levels began to steadily drop relative to those who were taking a placebo pill. The biggest drop occurred in the first few months, but the decrease continued over the course of the study.

After four years, participants in the metformin group had undergone a 19 percent relative reduction in their levels of the nutrient. They were 11.2 percent more likely than placebo participants to suffer from B12 insufficiency and 7.2 percent more likely to suffer from deficiency.

For every 8.9 patients treated with metformin, one would develop insufficient vitamin B12 levels. This increased risk remained after researchers adjusted for other risk factors including age, duration of diabetes, insulin dose, sex, smoking status and previous treatment with metformin.

"Our study shows that it is reasonable to assume harm will eventually occur in some patients with metformin-induced low vitamin B12 levels," the researchers wrote.

The researchers found that metformin seems to inhibit the intestine's absorption of vitamin B12. Fortunately, calcium supplements appear to reverse this effect.

Vitamin B12 is critical for maintaining nerve and red blood cell health. It can be found in animal products, nutritional yeast and fortified breakfast cereals. Symptoms of deficiency include anemia, fatigue, nerve damage and cognitive changes. Because similar symptoms often occur in diabetics and the elderly, deficiency may be hard to detect in such populations. Yet while B12 deficiency can carry severe consequences, it is relatively easy to correct with supplementation.

The researchers suggested that all patients taking metformin have their vitamin B12 levels tested regularly to avoid potentially severe consequences.

"Vitamin B-12 deficiency is preventable; therefore, our findings suggest that regular measurement of vitamin B-12 concentrations during long-term metformin treatment should be strongly considered." the researchers wrote.

Nearly 11 percent of the U.S. population, or 24 million people, suffer from diabetes. Of these 5.7 million are undiagnosed. In addition, 57 million people in the United States alone are estimated to be pre-diabetic, or at imminent risk of developing the disease.

Worldwide, an estimated 246 million people suffer from the disease. Prevalence is only expected to increase as the spreading Western diet and lifestyle lead to increasing rates of obesity.

Serious Dangers of Metformin

-**Lactic Acidosis** - is when lactic acid builds ups in the blood stream faster than it can be removed. Lactic acid is produced when oxygen levels in the body... Get emergency medical help if you have any of these symptoms of lactic acidosis:

weakness, increasing sleepiness, slow heart rate, cold feeling, muscle pain, shortness of breath, stomach pain, feeling light-headed, and fainting.

- **Anemia** - is a condition where there is a lower than normal number of red blood cells in the blood, usually measured by a decrease in the amount of hemoglobin....

-**Venous Insffeciency**-and poor blood circulation.

Other Side Effects:- decreased appetite- gas- heartburn- metallic taste in the mout-- mild stomachache- nausea/vomiting - weight loss- rash- diarrhea- flatulence- asthenia- indigestion- abdominal discomfort

Lifestyle changes win over metformin in lowering diabetes risk(From: www.lef.org):

Chapter IV

A study published in the February 7 2002 issue of the **New England Journal of Medicine** reported that results of a study of 3,234 individuals at risk for diabetes who were given either standard lifestyle recommendations along with a placebo or the drug metformin, or were prescribed an intensive lifestyle modification program consisting 150 minutes or more of exercise per week with the goal of at least 7% weight loss. Elevation of fasting and post-load plasma glucose concentrations qualified participants as being at risk of developing the disease. The trial was conducted at 27 centers and participants were followed up for an average of 2.8 years.

Those who received metformin, sold under the name Glucophage, received 850 mg twice per day. Standard lifestyle recommendations consisted of recommendations to follow the Food Guide Pyramid and a cholesterol-lowering diet to reduce their weight, and to increase exercise. The intensive lifestyle intervention involved a low calorie low fat diet, plus 150 minutes of exercise per week of moderate intensity, such as brisk walking.

During the follow up period, the incidence of diabetes was 31% lower in the group receiving metformin than the group receiving the placebo. However, in the lifestyle modification program, diagnoses of diabetes were 58% lower than those who received a placebo - 39% lower than the metformin group. Metformin and lifestyle intervention restored normal fasting glucose levels to a similar extent, but the lifestyle intervention more greatly improved post-load glucose levels. It was concluded that it should be possible to delay diabetes and its complications, reducing individual and public health burdens caused by this disease.

Insulin Dangers

Today, insulin is prescribed for both the Type I and Type II diabetics. Injectable insulin substitutes for the insulin that the body no longer produces. Of course, this treatment, while necessary for preserving the life of the Type I diabetic, is highly questionable when applied to the Type II diabetic.

It is important to note that neither insulin nor **any** of these oral hypoglycaemic agents exerts any curative action whatsoever on any type of diabetes. None of these medical strategies is designed to normalize the cellular uptake of glucose by the cells that need it to power their activity.

The prognosis with this orthodox treatment is increasing disability and early death from heart or kidney failure or the failure of some other vital organ.

Insulin Increases Mortality in Heart Failure Patients

UCLA researchers for the first time showed that advanced heart failure patients with diabetes who are treated with insulin faced a mortality rate four times higher than heart failure patients with diabetes treated with oral medications.

For full information about insulin dangers and side effects please read the book: INSULIN : OUR SILENT KILLER by Thomas Smith.

CHAPTER V

DIABETES AND H.PYLORI & HOW TO TREAT IT

A number of researchers noticed a relationship between diabetes and H.PYLORI presence in stomach ; one of them is JG SALUJA *Head; **Assoc. Prof. of Pathology; Medical College and Mumbadevi Homoeopathic Hospital and his team in Mumbai who concluded that incidence of H.PYLORI increases in diabetics **while our observations on diabetics** who followed our natural protocol for the last 10 years showed different results and gave different conclusions:

Some of diabetics who were on insulin together with Metformin informed us that they bought our herbal capsules and they used them with insulin and Metformin and they did not work and their blood sugar(FBS) remained over 400!!!!!! I asked them to test thyroid and stomach H.PYLORI!!! They told us that their doctors are asking why H.PYLORI?!!! There is no relationship between diabetes and H.PYLORI !!! We insisted on them to perform the test either by mouth breathing, blood test or stool and they did it and found a high concentration of H.PYLORI !!! and their thyroid tests were normal.Then they started a natural protocol to solve the H.PYLORI problem by taking MASTIC and Cinnamon for 3 weeks. During this period they noticed fast reduction in their blood sugar and they left metformin first then insulin gradually and kept taking our herbal capsules. They were astonished to see their blood sugar readings became less than 140 without medications in less than 3 weeks!!!!!

Our friend Dr.Bassam Khasawneh; M.D. in Yarmouk University started to ask his diabetics to perform the test and he found a high percentage diabetics have H.PYLORI in stomach!!!!!

Inflammation: The Root of Diabetes

More and more research pinpoints inflammation as a root cause of type 2 diabetes. Now it seems that inflammation even without obesity is the likely culprit. Research by scientists at the University of California, San Diego, and Switzerland's University of Fribourg discovered that inflammation provoked by immune cells called macrophages leads to insulin resistance and then to type 2 diabetes. Their research also showed that obesity without inflammation doesn't **result in insulin resistance.**

They made their discovery by working with mice, not humans. That gave them an advantage because they could use mice that lacked the macrophage JNK1.

Researchers at the University of California, San Diego (UCSD) School of Medicine have discovered that inflammation provoked by immune cells called macrophages leads to insulin resistance and Type 2 diabetes. Their discovery may pave the way to novel drug development to fight the epidemic of Type 2 diabetes. *Anti Inflammation Foods Reduce Type 2 Diabetes Up to 30%* Marc Y. Donath, MD, Clinic of Endocrinology and Diabetes, Department of Medicine, University Hospital, CH-8091 Zurich, Switzerland showed that the histology of islets from patients with type 2 diabetes displays an inflammatory process characterized by the presence of cytokines, apoptotic cells, immune cell infiltration, amyloid deposits, and eventually fibrosis. Inflammation caused to close the islet cells close partially hence does not help insulin to burn sugar the thing which leads to high sugar in blood.

A number of diabetics who follow our natural protocols when they feel a rise in their blood sugar they test H.PYLORI together with the tests related to inflammation such as WBC,ESR,C-REACTIVE PROTEIN and they usually take the natural anti-inflammatory products; Bee Propolis together with Azithromycin antibiotic for 3-6 days and they usually obtain lower sugar readings!!

We also noticed that any infection such as flu,cold, prostate, urinary tract, bladder, liver, mouth , vagina or stomach raises blood sugar and all types of infection are treated the same way mentioned above.

CHAPTER VI

DIABETES AND STRESS

Stress is defined as "a physical, chemical or emotional factor that causes physical or mental tension and may be a factor in disease causation." Several diseases can be caused or worsened by stress and diabetes is one of them.

Blood sugar levels are controlled mainly by two groups of hormones. The first group reduces blood sugar but insulin is the only member of this group. The second group called counter-regulatory hormones, opposes the action of insulin and increases the sugars.

There hormones include cortisol, adrenaline, noradrenaline, glucagon and growth hormone. Stress tends to increase the levels of these hormones, particularly cortisol, adrenaline and noradrenaline. If these levels are persistently elevated, this can precipitate diabetes in a predisposed individual or worsen it in someone who is already diabetic.

One of our patients   a 62-year-old lady from Jerusalem with abnormally high blood sugar levels of 350 mg/dl. Despite efforts to control her sugar levels with high doses of tablets, it remained above 300 mg/dl. But after she took our Relax-U aromatherapy perfume together with our relaxation advices and Vitamin B6 for 3 weeks her sugar levels began dropping and soon she was off medication as well.

It turned out that the lady's husband and son were creating problems for her, which put her under high stress. But once the problems ended, she was more relaxed and gradually her stress levels reduced and so did her sugar levels.

Jennifer Nelson wrote: (It's the nature of a fast-paced society, where numerous family, social, and work obligations can easily overpower your precious time and resources. But for people with diabetes , both physical and emotional stress can take a greater toll on health.

When you're stressed, your blood sugar levels rise. Stress hormones like epinephrine and cortisol kick in since one of their major functions is to raise blood sugar to help boost energy when it's needed most. Both physical and emotional stress can prompt an increase in these hormones, resulting in an increase in blood sugars.

People who aren't diabetic have compensatory mechanisms to keep blood sugar from swinging out of control. But in people with diabetes, those mechanisms are either lacking or blunted, so they can't keep a lid on blood sugar, says David Sledge, MD, medical director of diabetes management at The Ochsner Clinic Foundation in Baton Rouge, Louisiana.

"In diabetes, because of either an absolute lack of insulin, such as type 1 diabetes, or a relative lack of insulin, such as type 2, there isn't enough insulin to cope with these hormones, so blood sugar levels rise," says Richard Surwit, PhD, vice chairman of the department of psychiatry and behavioral sciences at Duke University Medical Center .

Anything upsetting like going through a breakup or being laid off is certainly emotionally draining. Being down with the flu or suffering from a urinary tract infection places physical stress on the body. It's generally these longer-term stressors that tax your system and have much more effect on blood sugar levels.

Stress-O-Meter

"The most important thing is to learn what it feels like when stress hormones are elevated," Sledge tells WebMD. "for some diabetic people, prolonged illness or distress will keep their blood sugar levels up for lengthy periods of time. Often insulin will be needed or adjusted during this period, so recognizing periods of stress is crucial for people with diabetes.

Since stress has virtually become a way of life, you may not even notice you're frazzled. A lot of people will identify stressors such as an illness in the family (something large) but may not recognize the stress of the holidays or a hectic time at work (something smaller or shorter in duration). Being in tune to your stress level and how you feel when the going gets tense is important. One good gauge is writing down your stress level in a journal each time you check your blood sugar. Many glucose meters have the capability to enter personal notes and data when you perform checks, or jot it down in a stress journal. "Once you begin recording stress levels, most people with diabetes figure out pretty quickly what makes their blood sugar go up," says Surwit.

One of the things that many people don't realize is the great impact that stress has on diabetes. Stress will cause the blood sugar generally to run quite a bit higher. This is related, we believe, to the fact that when we're under stress, our body puts out a lot of extra adrenaline into our bloodstream. And if anyone can think about a time when they've been worried or frightened, or otherwise injured, people get rapid heartbeat, they get shaky, they get tremors -- that's all the adrenaline fighting into

Chapter VI

the bloodstream. The other thing that that adrenaline does is that it jacks the blood sugar to a pretty high level. The idea is that should give us energy to deal with whatever harm or injury is done our way.

The body is not programmed though to take into account that some people have diabetes. So if the blood sugar's already high, here comes the stress, here comes an injury, the adrenaline shoots up, the blood sugar will shoot up even higher. So a lot of people will find out that whenever they have a very stressful event in their life, their sugar will go higher, and sometimes it takes a little time to figure that out, but there very, very clearly is a strong connection between those two things.

The harder part of the issue is how does one deal with stress, and I think there's as many answers to that as there are types of stress. I think first of all, knowledge that stress can do that is a very important thing. Certainly sitting down and thinking about, and reflecting on what are the stresses in my life -- are there any that are manageable, are there any that are correctible. Looking for some family support is very important. If there are some things out there that just seem insurmountable, going to a physician or seeking other outside help may be the right step to take).

The problem of stress may be compounded if for example a diabetic stressed woman gets a stressful heavy period!!! This may double stress and increase sugar level drastically!!!

How Stress Could be Managed?

Our protocol to manage stress consists of the following :

1-Diabetic should understand the equation between stress and diabetes and try to solve all problems that cause stress in his daily life.

2-It is recommended to take **Vitamin B6** and drink a calming tea such as **lemon balm tea** on daily basis.

3-It is recommended to have a sincere friend , to help him/her solve problems on continuous basis.

4-Get married if you are single:

(The 1858 groundbreaking study by British epidemiologist William Farr was one of the first scholarly works to suggest a "marriage advantage." The marriage advantage indicates that married people seem to have better health and live longer than unmarried people. Studies have shown that **a good marriage may help boost your immunity, <u>decrease stress levels</u>, lessen depression and anxiety, lower your blood pressure**

and reduce your risk of heart disease. And new research shows a happy marriage may even reduce arthritis pain).

In Holy Quran in Al-Rum Chapter we can find marriage a principal pillar of human life:

(030.021 And among His Signs is this, that He created for you mates from among yourselves, that ye may dwell in tranquillity with them, and He has put love and mercy between your (hearts): verily in that are Signs for those who reflect).

5-Read or listen Quran and natural music(**Delta Wave Music**)(Read about Alpha and Delta waves and their effects on stress ,diabetes and high blood pressure).

6-Have enough time to sleep.

7-Give yourself enough time of recreation on weekly basis.

8-Avoid foods/drinks that cause irritable colon (IBS) and indigestion

Laughter is the Best Medicine for Treatment of Venous Leg Ulcers?

Dr. Kristie Leong M.D. wrote on 18th March 2011:
Conventionally, doctors treat chronic venous leg ulcers by wrapping the leg in a compression bandage and having the patient keep it elevated. Some clinics use ultrasound therapy, but it isn't a very effective treatment according to a recent study in the British Medical Journal. In fact, this study concluded that laughter beats out ultrasound when it comes to the treatment of venous leg ulcers.
Why laughter? Laughter not only puts the patient in a positive mood, it stimulates movement of the diaphragm and increases blood flow to the legs, which is exactly what patients with chronic leg ulcers need. The researchers in this study point out that laughter is less expensive and more effective than ultrasound for speeding up the healing of chronic venous ulcers that can take many months to heal.

Comment: Laughter is not enough to heal venous leg/foot ulcer .Diabetics do need to take oral blood circulators together with natural wound/ulcer healing creams.

50

CHAPTER VII
DIABETES, ALCOHOL AND SMOKING

Alcoholism and Diabetes

There is a link between alcoholism and diabetes and it is often a dangerous one. In some cases, the link can lead to an early death if the person continues to drink. Diabetics who drink excessively will often experience progressing health problems. For some, diabetes alcoholism can be deadly since alcoholism has a very bad effect on liver and if we add the dangerous side effects of diabetes on heart ,kidney and blood circulation…etc the diabetic health becomes questionable!!!!

Diabetes alcoholism should be especially concerning for any diabetic who also has the following health issues. For these individuals, any amount of alcohol can be dangerous:

- Any type of damage to the nerves in either the arms or legs.
- Any sign of diabetic eye disease.
- Any sign of increased blood pressure.
- Any sign of increased triglycerides.
- Any sign of ESR OR CRP increased test values.
- Any sign of increased kidney functions values.
- Any sign of increased liver ezymes.

One of the most common issues with alcoholism and diabetes is nerve damage. It should be noted that any amount of drinking can lead to nerve damage, in both diabetics and non-diabetics. For diabetics, however, who also have some form of nerve damage, drinking will often increase the pain, tingling, numbness, or burning sensations that are usually associated with diabetic nerve damage.

Because of the chemical composition of alcohol, those who have high triglycerides should avoid all forms of alcohol, as consumption of even small amounts will increase the levels of triglycerides in the blood system especially if the diabetic does not have a daily sport or walking program.

If You Take Medication

Alcoholism will also cause severe problems for those who are taking either oral medications or insulin shots for their diabetes. In these cases, drinking can lead to low blood sugar levels. Under normal circumstances, when blood sugar levels drop off, the liver will produce glucose to help compensate for the drop. Alcohol consumption, however, will block glucose production from the liver. The liver will continue to avoid producing glucose until the alcohol has been cleared from the body. This is one of the main reasons persons suffering from alcoholism and diabetes should avoid consuming alcohol.

For those diabetics who are allowed light drinking, the American Diabetes Association recommends never to consume alcohol on an empty stomach. These individual should only drink after they have had something to eat. They should also eat something before they go to bed after drinking. This can help to prevent a low blood sugar event.

For Type 2 diabetics, those who can control their diabetes with diet and exercise, instead of medication, drinking alcohol will usually be less of a risk factor for low blood sugar events.

The Best Advice

It is a myth, and a dangerous one, for all diabetics to believe that they can have a few drinks and do so safely. The truth is simple: some diabetics cannot drink alcohol at any level and be safe. Knowing where you stand on this important issue is vital to maintaining good health. It is also important to remember that many of the symptoms associated with this problem will not be felt immediately, thus making the person believe that they are all right while they are drinking.

Those concerned with alcoholism and diabetes should consult with their doctor before drinking. This is the only way to know for sure if a problem may occur. Once the consult is finished, persons with diabetes alcoholism issues should follow the advice given to the letter. Some health issues, especially the most dangerous ones, can occur very rapidly if their doctor's advice is ignored.

Chapter VII

Can Alcoholism Cause Diabetes?

Alcoholism is classified as a disease that causes the body to become dependent on frequent alcohol consumption. Alcoholism can lead to many adverse health conditions and may even cause diabetes to develop in some individuals. Those individuals who already have diabetes may also suffer additional adverse affects of consuming excess alcohol.

Pancreatitis

o **According to the Mayo Clinic**, drinking alcohol excessively can lead to pancreatitis. Pancreatitis can damage the pancreas, so it is no longer able to secrete adequate amounts of insulin to control blood sugar. This can cause diabetes to develop.

Glucose Intolerance

o Alcohol consumption may also lead to glucose intolerance and eventually lead to diabetes.

o Impairs Insulin Response

o Excessive drinking may cause the body to stop responding appropriately to insulin. Over time, this can cause diabetes to develop.

o Raises Blood Sugar

o Drinking alcohol excessively can increase the secretion of hormones that raise blood sugar levels.

Weight Gain

o Being obese puts individuals at a greater risk of developing diabetes. Drinking excessive high-calorie alcoholic drinks may lead to obesity and increase this risk.

References: Mayo Clinic Site about : Alcohol and Diabetes and Alcoholism.com

How to Quit Drinking?

o -Learn more from health sites about alcoholism dangers on your health especially impotence , infertility and liver damage.

o -Learn more about social problems created as a result of alcoholism.

o -Try to take Fo-Ti dietary supplement or FO-TI Tea on daily basis

Smoking and Diabetes

American Diabetes Association summarizes the relationship between smoking and diabetes by the following statement:

(It is no secret that smoking is bad for your health. Smoking hurts your lungs and your heart. It lowers the amount of oxygen that gets to your organs, raises your bad cholesterol, and raises your blood pressure. All of these can raise your risk of heart attack or stroke).

*In an article in The **Daily Mail Newspaper** a number of researchers explained how smoking causes more than 50 diseases ; lung ,skin and mouth cancers, heart disorder,high blood pressure,stroke,infertility,impotence....etc.*

Smoking During Pregnancy Linked to Gestational Diabetes Risk

BETHESDA, MD — January 28, 2005 (Woman who smoke have a greater chance of developing gestational diabetes, a form of diabetes that first occurs during pregnancy, a new study suggests (Am J Epidemiol. 2004 Dec 15; 160(12): 1205–13). Gestational diabetes can lead to preeclampsia, a condition involving high blood pressure, protein in the urine, fluid retention, and swelling in the hands and feet. These women may also deliver very large babies (fetal macrosomia). In some cases, they continue to have diabetes (type 2 diabetes mellitus) in later years.)

Like drinking too much alcohol or doing drugs, smoking is also very harmful to your health. It can cause serious health conditions including cancer, heart disease, stroke and gum disease. It can also cause eye diseases that can lead to blindness. Smoking can make it harder for a woman to get pregnant.

Not only is smoking harmful to you, it's also harmful to your baby during pregnancy. When you smoke during pregnancy, your baby is exposed to dangerous chemicals like nicotine, carbon monoxide and tar.

Chapter VII ─────────────

These chemicals can lessen the amount of oxygen that your baby gets. Oxygen is very important for helping your baby grow healthy. Smoking can also damage your baby's lungs.

Secondhand Smoke Breathing in someone else's smoke is also harmful. Secondhand smoke during pregnancy can cause a baby to be born at low birth weight. Secondhand smoke is also dangerous to young children. Babies exposed to secondhand smoke:

- o -Are more likely to die from SIDS (Sudden Infant Death Syndrome)
- o -Are at greater risk for asthma, bronchitis, pneumonia, ear infections, respiratory symptoms
- o -May experience slow lung growth

Why Smoking increases the Risk of Diabetes?

Smoking has the same vasoconstrictive effects on diabetic veins similar to the ones caused by diabetes and some diabetes drugs. **Hisako Fushimi et al from** Department of Medicine, Sumitomo Hospital, Osaka, Japan(Diabetes Research and Clinical Practice,vol 16,1992,pp191-195) found a direct vasoconstrictive effects on diabetic veins the thing which doubles the risk of diabetes.

Passive Smoking

One of the main reasons for introducing a public smoking ban is to protect people from the risk of passive smoking. Read the reports and make up your own mind on the danger.

NEW YORK, March 11, (RTRS): Cigarette smoke is tied to a higher risk of type 2 diabetes, formerly known as adult-onset diabetes, for both smokers and the people around them, a study said.And the more secondhand smoke people are exposed to, the greater their risk of the disease, which results from insulin resistance — in which cells fail to use insulin properly — sometimes combined with an absolute insulin deficiency, according to the study, published in "Diabetes

Care.'"'Accumulating evidence has identified a positive association between active smoking and the risk of diabetes, but previous studies had limited information on passive smoking or changes in smoking behavior over time," wrote John Forman at Brigham and Women's hospital in Boston, who led the study.The study followed 100,000 women over 24 years.

<u>How to Quit Smoking:</u>

1-Try to see your black lung CT-SCAN and compare it with ones of non-smokers which look rosey!!!

2-Try to count all economical and social side effects surrounding your life.

3-Try to drink the herbal juice of rocket vegetable juice on daily basis.

4-The smokers who used our pleasant **Bye Bye Smoking Perfume** in their nose daily quit smoking within four weeks gradually without any withdrawal side effects.

CHAPTER VIII
DIABETES AND RACE

It's estimated that more than 23 million, or nearly 11 percent, of U.S. adults have type 2 diabetes. The most important risk factors for type 2 diabetes include older age, obesity, family history of diabetes and race -- with black, Hispanic and Native Americans at higher risk than whites in the U.S. The extent to which specific nutrients in the diet might affect diabetes risk remains unclear.

Some studies showed that: For every six white Americans who have diabetes, 10 African Americans have diabetes.

African Americans with diabetes are more likely to develop diabetes complications and experience greater disability from the complications than white Americans with diabetes.

How Many African Americans Have Diabetes?

These studies show the prevalence for African American men and women based on the most recent national studies.

About one-third of total diabetes cases are undiagnosed among African Americans. This is similar to the proportion for other racial/ethnic groups in the United States.

National health surveys during the past 35 years show that the percentage of the African American population that has been diagnosed with diabetes is increasing dramatically. The surveys in 1976-80 and in 1988-94 measured fasting plasma glucose and thus allowed an assessment of the prevalence of undiagnosed diabetes as well as of previously diagnosed diabetes. In 1976-80, total diabetes prevalence in African Americans age 40-74 years was 8.9 percent; in 1988-94, total prevalence had increased to 18.2 percent--a doubling of the rate in just 12 years.

Prevalence in African Americans is much higher than in white Americans. Among those age 40-74 years in the 1988-94 survey, the rate was 11.2 percent for whites, but was 18.2 percent for blacks--diabetes prevalence in blacks is 1.6 times the prevalence in whites.

Genetic Risk Factors

The common finding that "diabetes runs in families" indicates that there is a strong genetic component to type 1 and type 2 diabetes. Many scientists are now conducting research to determine the genes that cause diabetes. For type 1 diabetes, certain genes related to immunology have been implicated. For type 2 diabetes, there seem to be diabetes genes that determine insulin secretion and insulin resistance. Some researchers believe that African Americans inherited a "thrifty gene" from their African ancestors. Years ago, this gene enabled Africans, during "feast and famine" cycles, to use food energy more efficiently when food was scarce. Today, with fewer such cycles, the thrifty gene that developed for survival may instead make the person more susceptible to developing type 2 diabetes.

Obesity

Overweight is a major risk factor for type 2 diabetes. The NHANES surveys found that overweight is increasing in the United States, both in adolescents and in adults. Studies support these data and also shows that African American adults have substantially higher rates of obesity than white Americans.

In addition to the overall level of obesity, the location of the excess weight is also a risk factor for type 2 diabetes. Excess weight carried above the waist is a stronger risk factor than excess weight carried below the waist. African Americans have a greater tendency to develop upper-body obesity, which increases their risk of diabetes.

Although African Americans have higher rates of obesity, researchers do not believe that obesity alone accounts for their higher prevalence of diabetes. Even when compared with white Americans with the same levels of obesity, age, and socioeconomic status, African Americans still have higher rates of diabetes. Other factors, yet to be understood, appear to be responsible.

Chapter VIII

Physical Activity

Regular physical activity is a protective factor against type 2 diabetes and, conversely, lack of physical activity is a risk factor for developing diabetes. Researchers suspect that a lack of exercise is one factor contributing to the high rates of diabetes in African Americans. In the NHANES III survey, 50 percent of black men and 67 percent of black women reported that they participated in little or no leisure time physical activity.

How Does Diabetes Affect African-American Young People?

African American children seem to have lower rates of type 1 diabetes than white American children. Researchers tend to agree that genetics probably makes type 1 diabetes less common among children with African ancestry compared with children of European ancestry.

Comments:

1-The above studies covered Afro-Americans compared to White Americans and it should cover original African people in order to arrive at justified scientific conclusions.

2- Other major factors such as obesity, types of food and drinks ,poverty, stress ...etc should be taken into consideration if we want to generalize the results of the above studies.

References :

1. American Diabetes Association. Report of the Expert Committee on the Diagnosis and Classification of Diabetes Mellitus. Diabetes Care, Vol. 20, p. 1183-1197, 1997.

2. Harris MI, Flegal KM, Cowie CC, et al. Prevalence of Diabetes, Impaired Fasting Glucose, and Impaired Glucose Tolerance in U.S. Adults: The Third National Health and Nutrition Examination Survey, 1988-94. Diabetes Care Vol. 21, p. 518-524, 1998.

3. Tull ES, Roseman JM. Diabetes in African Americans. Chapter 31 in Diabetes in America. 2nd Edition (NIH Publication No. 95-1468, pp. 613-630

4. Harris MI. Unpublished data from the Third National Health and Nutrition Examination Survey, 1988-94.

5. Jiang X, Srinivasan SR, Radhakrishnamurthy B, Dalferes ER, Berenson GS: Racial (black-white) differences in insulin secretion and clearance in adolescents: the Bogalusa heart study. Pediatrics 97:357-360, 1996.

6. Kuzmarski RJ, Flegal KM, Campbell SM, Johnson CL: Increasing prevalence of overweight among US adults. The National Health and Nutrition Examination Surveys, 1960 to 1991. JAMA 272:205-211, 1994.

7. Troiano RP, Flegal KM, Kuczmarski RJ, Campbell SM, Johnson CL: Overweight prevalence and trends for children and adolescents. Arch Pediatr Adolesc Med 149:1085-1091, 1995.

8. Crespo CJ, Keteyian SJ, Heath GW, Sempos CT: Leisure-time physical activity among US adults. Arch Intern Med 156:93-98, 1996.

CHAPTER IX
DIABETES AND METABOLIC SYNDROME X

Insulin Resistance Syndrome (IRS) (also called Metabolic Syndrome and previously called Syndrome X)

What is insulin resistance?

The term insulin resistance is used when a person makes insulin but resists the effects of the insulin. That is, the normal action of insulin (carbohydrate metabolism) in the body is compromised.

When a person is insulin resistant, their cells do not respond to a normal secretion of insulin, and requires a higher level (more) insulin to move blood glucose (sugar) out of the blood stream and into cells.

A person that is with insulin resistance can still have normal fasting blood glucose (blood sugar) levels and after meals, as well as "pass" an oral glucose tolerance test (OGTT). In order to maintain these normal glucose levels, a person will overproduce insulin. Elevated insulin level is called "hyperinsulinemia."

What is insulin resistance? It is a metabolic disorder that increases the chances of developing type 2 diabetes and heart disease.

It may exist without other problems, especially when caught early. But left untreated, insulin resistance typically gets worse and other symptoms begin to appear. When a combination of certain factors exist a person may be diagnosed with Insulin Resistance Syndrome.

Symptoms of Overproducing Insulin

To be diagnosed as insulin resistant, your doctor will need to run certain lab tests. However, a patient often has signs and symptoms that occur before a diagnosis is made. These include:

- hypoglycemia (low blood glucose levels), but levels may also be high or normal
- mild hyperglycemia (high blood glucose levels), but levels may also be low or normal
- food cravings, especially for carbohydrates
- weight gain, often rapid, and prone to carry excess weight around the waist

- sleep disruption
- lethargy
- hirsutism in women (excessive facial hair or developing male hair pattern traits)
- skin tags
- acne
- acanthosis nigricans
- alopecia areata (scalp and/or body hair loss)
- depression and mood swings
- changes in the menstrual cycle
- yeast infections
- bloating
- often have high LDL (bad) cholesterol and low HDL (good) cholesterol
- high levels of triglycerides
- high blood pressure (hypertension)
- Side Effects of Overproducing Insulin
- Over production of insulin can aggravate or trigger other problems including infertility, weight gain, bloating, poor lipid profiles, hormonal imbalances, cosmetic problems (hair loss, hirsutism, skin tags, acanthosis nigricans), and contribute to more serious health risks like high blood pressure, heart problems, and an increased risk of developing diabetes, and gestational diabetes during pregnancy.
- A pancreas that continually over produces insulin may also, over time, wear out, in which case a patient usually will need to take insulin.

Causes of Insulin Resistance

- Many things can contribute to insulin resistance including obesity, an inactive lifestyle, high levels of caffeine, certain medications, and underlying medical problems. Other things that can contribute to insulin resistance include pregnancy and hormonal imbalances (i.e. Hashimoto's thyroiditis or other hypothyroid problems, and

Chapter IX ─────────

polycystic ovarian syndrome (PCOS)).

- Since insulin resistance, and many of the disorders associated with this condition tend to run in families, genes also play a role in the development of insulin resistance. But it is important to note that studies show simply having the genetic predisposition for insulin resistance or type 2 diabetes is not enough to cause onset. Many people carry the risk genes for either type 2 or type 1 diabetes and still do not end up becoming diabetic. Some sort of environmental trigger usually contributes to the onset of diabetes. In the case of type 2 diabetes the environmental trigger is an unhealthy lifestyle including poor eating habits, too little activity, obesity, and smoking.

- So remember that, even if you have family members that are insulin resistant, obese, or have diabetes, it should be considered a warning sign of potential risk for you, but following a healthy lifestyle will go a long way towards reducing the risk that you too, will develop metabolic disorders.

Insulin Resistance in Diabetes Types 1 and 2

For persons with diabetes, insulin resistance is more commonly seen in type 2 patients, but sometimes those that are type 1 can also have, or develop, a true resistance to insulin. For those that take insulin injections, repeatedly using the same injection site can cause damage to surrounding tissues that makes the area less sensitive to insulin. Rotating injection and cannula sites is important to help prevent this localized insulin resistance.

A syndrome is different from a disease: To be diagnosed with a disease a person must meet a specific list of symptom or medical criteria. To be classified as having a syndrome, a person may have only some of the characteristics associated with that particular syndrome.

Insulin Resistance Syndrome is a combination of problems. It is diagnosed when a patient has at least three factors identified as part of IRS. (See "Diagnosing Insulin Resistance Syndrome," below).

Diagnosing Insulin Resistance & Insulin Resistance Syndrome (IRS) :To be certain whether or not a person is insulin resistant, a normal glucose tolerance test, or morning fasting blood glucose test is helpful and should be done, however is not sufficient to diagnosed or rule out insulin resistance. Along with blood glucose, fasting insulin levels should also be checked. Persons that are insulin resistant may have normal,or elevated blood glucose levels (or sometimes may be hypoglycemic, having low blood glucose levels). But all persons with insulin resistance will have higher than normal levels of insulin regardless of blood glucose levels.

Several measures of insulin can be used to determine insulin resistance, although, one is not practical for most people:

- **Euglycemia clamp** - this test is both expensive and complicated, and most often used in scientific research.

- **Fasting insulin levels** - a simple blood test after overnight fasting (no food or drink except water for at least 8 hours) can measure insulin levels.

- **Insulin Resistance Index (IRI)** - this is a comparison between glucose levels and insulin levels. Using the IRI as a measurement for insulin resistance:

Insulin Resistance Index Values

Less than 2.67	Normal values
Between 2.93 and 3.12	Typically found in persons that are obese and may indicate insulin resistance
Above 3.22	Indicates prediabetes or type 2 diabetes

A diagnosis of Insulin Resistance Syndrome (IRS) may be made when any three of the following criteria are met:

-Prediabetes

-Polycystic Ovarian Syndrome (PCOS)

-Fasting Glucose of ≥ 112 mg/dL, or current use of diabetic medication

Abdominal obesity (especially apple shaped body) with a waist circumference:
Women >35 inches

Chapter IX ────────────────────────

Men   > 40 inches

High Blood Pressure hypotension):
Systolic   ≥ 130 mm HG or
Diastolic   ≥ 85 mm HG or
current use of blood pressure medication

Low HDL Cholesterol ("good" cholesterol)
Women   < 50
Men   < 40, or

Elevated Triglycerides
≥150 mg/dL

Treatment for Insulin Resistance and Insulin Resistance Syndrome

Insulin Resistance (IR) - IR can be treated through <u>Lifestyle management</u> including weight loss, and exercise. Persons who are IR usually benefit from a diet low in processed carbohydrates and fat, or low-glycemic index plans. They may gain weight even on moderate- to low-calorie diets if they are high in carbohydrates because consumption of carbohydrates (simple or complex) can trigger over production of insulin -- a fat storing hormone.

Sometimes insulin sensitizing oral medications like Glucophage are also prescribed. It should be noted that weight loss and exercise have been shown to be overall more effective at stopping the progression of, and reversing insulin resistance, than medication.

Insulin Resistance Syndrome - Many aspects of IRS can be treated through <u>Lifestyle management</u> including weight loss and exercise. Persons who are insulin resistant usually benefit from a diet low in processed carbohydrate and fat, or from following low-glycemic index plans. They may gain weight even on moderate- to low-calorie diets that are high in carbohydrates because consumption of carbohydrates (simple or complex) can trigger over production of insulin -- a fat storing hormone. Sometimes oral medications are prescribed for insulin sensitizing, or for other symptoms like high cholesterol or blood pressure.

It should be noted that weight loss and exercise have been shown to be over all, more effective at stopping the progression of, and reversing insulin resistance which is at the heart of other problems associated with IRS.

To see if you may need to lose weight, read about "<u>Body Mass</u>

Other Metabolic Disorders that may be Associated with Insulin Resistance

Other conditions may cause, be exacerbated, or result from insulin resistance. It is important for your doctor to take a complete medical history for you, and for family members as some disorders can be hereditary in nature. Be sure to tell your doctor if any family members have autoimmune disorders, metabolic disorders, or other serious health problems like cancer, heart disease, or high blood pressure or cholesterol.

In addition to the potential for diabetes, other disorders that may also be present with either insulin resistance, or with IRS include:

- Addison's Disease
- Asthma and Allergies
- Celiac Disease (Sprue)
- Cushing's Syndrome
- Cyclic Vomiting Syndrome
- Cystic Fibrosis (which can lead to CF related diabetes)
- Eating Disorders
- Fibromyalgia Syndrome
- Frozen Shoulder (though more common in persons with diabetes)
- Hashimoto's Thyroiditis
- Hemochromatosis (also called "Iron Overload" or "Bronze Diabetes")
- Infertility
- Irritable Bowel Syndrome
- Polycystic Ovarian Syndrome (PCOS)
- Weight Gain
- Weight Loss
- **Prognosis for Insulin Resistance and Insulin Resistance Syndrome**
- Since insulin resistance may be the result of poor lifestyle habits

66

Chapter IX ————————————————

it can often be completely reversed or halted from further progression by simply adopting more healthy eating and an exercise plan. Even when there is another underlying disorder that requires additional treatment, with proper medical care and a healthy lifestyle, most disorders can be managed very effectively.

- Insulin resistance, just one aspect of IRS can often be completely reversed or halted from further progression with lifestyle changes, although sometimes insulin sensitizing drugs may be prescribed. But if let untreated, insulin resistance can develop into more complex medical problems including pred iabetes, and even lead to the onset of type 2 diabetes. It may also be a triggering factor in other medical problems and disorders. And, both IR and IRS can also worsen the symptoms and increase the likelihood of complications from other disorders sometimes associated with IRS, including Hashimoto's Thyroiditis, Addison's Disease, and Cushing's Syndrome.

- Women that have PCOS typically experience worsening of their symptoms of PCOS when insulin resistance is not addressed medically and through lifestyle changes. This not only has cosmetic impact (acne, excess facial hair, scalp hair loss, etc.) but can also have a strong, negative impact on fertility and increases the risk of serious complications of PCOS including diabetes, heart disease, and cancer.

- A hallmark of IRS is often poor lipid profiles which can result in complications and health problems from high blood pressure, low HDL cholesterol and high LDL cholesterol and/or triglycerides. Risks include stroke and heart attack, and an increased risk of certain types of cancers.

- The upside is that, for the most part, unlike diabetes, insulin resistance can be reversed and controlled. See your doctor as soon as possible if you suspect you have any of the symptoms or signs of insulin resistance

CHAPTER X
DIABETES,TRIGLYCERIDES, CHOLESTEROL AND OBESITY

High Triglycerides Trigger Metabolic Dysfunction and Disease Risk

Triglycerides account for about 99 percent of the fat stored in our bodies. These triglyceride- fats serve as the most important source of long-term energy for the body, since they are stored in a much denser form than starches or muscle proteins. Formation of fat requires the presence of insulin. Triglyceride in fat is converted to energy between meals and overnight, or any time when we are fasting or insulin levels are low. Fat cells have a tremendous storage capacity, which may contribute to obesity. With extended fasting or absolute insulin deficiency, the liver converts fat breakdown products to ketones.

High triglyceride levels in the blood tend to coexist with low levels of HDL ("good") cholesterol, contributing to a condition called diabetic dyslipidemia. The third component of this "dangerous trio" is a tendency for patients with this condition to have the small, dense, undesirable (more atherogenic) type of LDL cholesterol in their blood (even though their LDL cholesterol level may be normal).

The combination of high triglycerides, low HDL and central obesity are the hallmarks of the metabolic syndrome, which occurs in 80 percent of people with type 2 diabetes. The frightening significance of this combination of risk factors is the marked incidence in these people of premature death from heart disease.

Our modern diet is laced with processed junk foods packed with excess sugar and refined carbohydrates which lead to large blood sugar spikes and ultimately to metabolic disorder. The body deals with high blood sugar levels by converting to triglycerides, and then into stored body fat. As this process continues over the course of a lifetime, systemic inflammation increases and the devastating effects of metabolic syndrome (high blood pressure and blood sugar, obesity and insulin resistance) dramatically increase the risk of heart disease and diabetes.

One reason for body cells to fail to take up glucose (blood sugar) properly is

- lack of insulin, common in type 1 diabetes, also called insulin-dependent or juvenile diabetes) or

- insulin resistance, in which the body can't use insulin efficiently, common in type 2 diabetes, sometimes referred to as maturity-onset diabetes or noninsulin-dependent diabetes mellitus (NIDDM), or
- insulin resistance syndrome, also called metabolic syndrome X or pre-diabetes syndrome, or
- all the above.
- High blood triglycerides levels - over 199 mg/dL, or 2.3 mmol/L - are a common symptom of pre-diabetes. Furthermore, you will be considered pre-diabetic if your fasting blood sugar level is between 110 mg/dL and 125 mg/dL (diabetes is formally diagnosed at 126 mg/dL).
- Findings of a recent research shows significant role of high triglycerides in the progression of diabetic neuropathy.

Findings of a recent research shows significant role of high triglycerides in the progression of diabetic neuropathy.

"High triglyceride levels the most common feature of the lipid disorder found in patients with type 2 diabetes" says Rodica Pop-Busui, M.D., Ph.D., one of the study's authors and an assistant professor in the metabolism, endocrinology and diabetes division of the Department of Internal Medicine at the U-M Medical School .

The study also found that there is a tight link between cardiovascular disease and peripheral neuropathy in patients with diabetes.

The study also found that same lipid particles contributing to the progression of clogging of arteries are very important in peripheral neuropathy.

The study further confirms that elevated triglyceride is a key factor in the progression of diabetic neuropathy . High triglycerides and diabetes makes a dangerous combination and may results into complications like diabetic neuropathy.

Two studies recently reported on the connection between high triglycerides and diabetic related amputations. Published recently online in **Diabetes** (2009) and **Lancet** (2009), one linked high triglycerides to diabetic neuropathy, (the leading cause of amputations in diabetics) while the other study showed that controlling high levels of triglycerides helped reduce the number of amputations.

Chapter X

Increased Waistline and High Triglycerides Increase Risk of Heart Disease

Information published in the *Canadian Medical Association Journal* found that increased waist size and triglyceride levels were associated with the highest risk for coronary artery disease. While both factors were found to increase heart disease risk, the combination of the two significantly raised the likelihood of developing coronary artery disease. High triglycerides contribute to thickening of the arterial walls which greatly increases the incidence of stroke, heart attack and congestive heart failure.

Increased triglyceride levels are indicative of a metabolic fat disorder and are implicated in nearly two-thirds of all coronary heart disease cases. Until recently, high triglycerides have been largely ignored by many medical professionals because they don't respond well to prescription drugs. Sadly, most physicians know that if dietary and lifestyle changes are needed to treat a condition, compliance by the patient will be minimal.

Diabetes and Cholesterol Link

High cholesterol levels are as serious as high blood pressure, whether you are diabetic or non-diabetic. Heart disease and stroke, both of which have been linked to high cholesterol in both men and women, are two of the leading causes of death for diabetics.

How does diabetes affect cholesterol?

Diabetes tends to lower "good" cholesterol levels and raise triglyceride and "bad" cholesterol levels, which increases the risk for heart disease and stroke. This common condition is called diabetic dyslipidemia.

"Diabetic dyslipidemia means your lipid profile is going in the wrong direction," said Richard Nesto, M.D., a spokesperson for the American Heart Association. "It's a deadly combination that puts patients at risk for premature coronary heart disease and atherosclerosis — where the arteries become clogged with accumulated fat and other substances."

Studies show a link between insulin resistance, which is a precursor to type 2 diabetes, and diabetic dyslipidemia, atherosclerosis and blood vessel disease. These conditions can develop even before diabetes is diagnosed.

According to (Reuters) - People on cholesterol-lowering statins are 9 percent more likely to develop diabetes, but this small absolute risk is outweighed by the drugs' heart-protecting properties,

71

researchers said on Wednesday.

Bad Cholesterol (LDL) Link with Diabetes There are various factors which contribute to increased LDL levels, such as smoking, obesity, sedentary life, family history, hypertension. These factors contribute to diabetes onset. Thus, diabetics have more chances to develop heart disease. In recent studies it was discovered that bad cholesterol is one of the causes of type II diabetes.

Obesity Increases Risk of Diabetes

For **men** with diabetes and the apple figure (**with excess weight in the middle**) the risk for heart disease goes up two and a half times, for **women** with diabetes and this shape it rises eightfold.

Why is the apple figure risky?

Fat cells located in the abdomen release fat into the blood more easily than fat cells found elsewhere. Release of fat begins 3 to 4 hours after the last meal compared to many more hours for other fat cells.

This easy release shows up as higher triglyceride and free fatty acid levels. Free fatty acids themselves cause insulin resistance. It is estimated that one out of every four people in the U.S., or 80 million Americans, have insulin resistance and they are more prone to heart disease, even though they may never actually develop diabetes.

Excess cardiac risks found with an apple figure include:

- higher blood triglycerides levels
- lower HDL-"good" (protective) cholesterol
- higher blood pressure
- type 2 diabetes, and
- kidney disease.

Researchers from Saint Louis University School of Medicine, Missouri have found that high triglycerides block leptin - a hormone secreted by our fat cells - from getting into the brain by impairing its transportation system (*Diabetes, 2004: May*).As a result, leptin cannot do its work in turning off feeding and burning calories.

In other words, high triglycerides make the brain "think" the body is starving so we keep eating and... gaining weight. This is probably one of the reasons why so many people are becoming obese. By lowering triglycerides then, we could help the body's own leptin to work better so we could get skinnier avoiding heart problems, cancer and diabetes - common chronic diseases linked to obesity.

CHAPTER XI
DIABETES AND IMMUNITY
TYPE I DIABETES AND IMMUNITY

Abner L. Notkins,from National Institute of Health, in Maryland wrote about the link between type 1 diabetes and immune system:

(Type 1 diabetes is due to a deficiency of insulin as a result of destruction of the pancreatic β cells. At the time of clinical symptoms, 60–80% of the β cells are destroyed. Cells secreting glucagon, somatostatin, and pancreatic polypeptide are generally preserved but may be redistributed within the islets. Insulitis, an inflammatory infiltrate containing large numbers of mononuclear cells and CD8 T cells, typically occurs around or within individual islets.

The cause of β cell destruction remained an enigma for years, but two discoveries in the 1970s provided the basis for the current thinking about the disease. The first was a strong linkage of type 1 diabetes to the highly polymorphic HLA class II immune recognition molecules

Hundreds of studies have now been carried out in laboratories around the world to determine the relationship between autoantibodies to GAD/IA-2/insulin and type 1 diabetes . Approximately 70–80% of newly diagnosed type 1 diabetes patients have autoantibodies to GAD65. Nearly the same number or slightly less have autoantibodies to IA-2. Overall, fewer patients appear to have insulin autoantibodies, but this is due to a pronounced age effect: children with newly diagnosed type 1 diabetes have a markedly higher frequency of autoantibodies to insulin than teenagers or young adults . Some patients carry autoantibodies to only one of the major autoantigens, but others may react to all three. In newly diagnosed subjects, up to 90% have autoantibodies to one or more of these antigens. The percent positivity depends on a variety of factors, including not only the age of the subjects, but also the duration of the disease and, in some cases, their ethnic origins

Environmental factors such as pathogens, toxins, drugs, and food components have long been thought to contribute to the pathogenesis of type 1 diabetes, with viruses being the leading environmental candidate . Animal studies have shown that viruses can infect pancreatic β cells and that the development of diabetes is dependent upon both the genetic background of the animal and the viral strain. Indeed, a single amino acid substitution within the virus can determine whether or not diabetes develops .

Based on the presence of autoantibodies and a strong HLA linkage, type 1 diabetes is now classified as a chronic autoimmune disease. Many issues, however, remain unresolved. Although autoantibodies to GAD65, IA-2, and insulin are clearly markers for this disease, it is not known whether they contribute to pathogenesis or are simply the response to an existing underlying destructive process. Based on extensive studies in animal models, it is thought that it is the cell-mediated immune response that is actually responsible for the destruction of β cells.

The cause of β cell destruction remained an enigma for years, but two discoveries in the 1970s provided the basis for our current thinking about the disease. The first was a strong linkage of type 1 diabetes to the highly polymorphic HLA class II immune recognition molecules.)

Joseph F. Plouffe et al f from the University of Michigan Medical Center, Ann Arbor in a recent study summarized their findings about the relationship between immunity and diabetes as follows:

Cell-mediated immunity was evaluated in patients with diabetes mellitus by delayed hypersensitivity skin tests and in vitro lymphocyte transformations. Only 44% of diabetic patients had skin test reactivity to *Candida* antigen, compared with 88% of normal controls . **Insulin-dependent diabetic** (Type I Diabetes) patients had abnormally low lymphocyte transformation responses .This defect was not corrected by culturing the cells in nondiabetic plasma. Type I diabetics with persistent hyperglycemia (fasting serum glucose level, >200 mg/dl) had lower levels of transformation than did the same type patients with fasting serum glucose levels less than 150 mg/dl. Lymphocytes from two Type I patients with poor lymphocyte transformation responses had marked improvement. Seven Type I patients were studied serially over 12 months. Lymphocyte transformation responses in four of these patients improved coincidentally with a change in the level of fasting hyperglycemia from >200 to <150 mg/dl. The other three Type I patients with consistent fasting serum glucose levels of >200 mg/dl had poor lymphocyte transformation responses. Diabetic patients have

Chapter XI ────────────────

demonstrable defects in lymphocyte function which improved in a small number of patients with reduction in the level of fasting hyperglycemia.

TYPE II DIABETES AND IMMUNITY

A new study by researchers at Stanford University and the University of Toronto, however, suggests that type 2 diabetes may involve immune system abnormalities after all. The researchers also found that blood samples of people with type 2 diabetes contained antibodies against some of their own proteins. In other words, their immune systems have turned on them.

Doctors believe that the haemoglobin A1C or HBA1C the cumulative reading of blood sugar for 3 months is correlated to immunity; and blood sugar readings and HBA1C are directly proportional .Higher HBA1C reflects higher blood sugar and likelihood for weaker immunity.

EFFECT OF DIABETES ON IMMUNITY

Research led by the Warwick Medical School at the University of Warwick has found that unhealthy glucose levels in patients with diabetes can cause significantly more problems for the body than just the well-known symptoms of the disease such as kidney damage and circulation problems. The raised glucose can also form what can be described as a sugar coating that can effectively smother and block the mechanisms our bodies use to detect and fight bacterial and fungal infections.

In diabetes, patients suffer a higher risk of chronic bacterial and fungal infections but until now little has been known about the mechanisms involved. Now new research led by Dr Daniel Mitchell at the University of Warwick's Medical School has found a novel relationship between high glucose and the immune system in humans. The researchers have found that specialized receptors that recognize molecules associated with bacteria and fungi become "blind" when glucose levels rise above healthy levels. The new research may also help explain why diabetic complications can also include increased risk of viral infections such as flue, and also inflammatory conditions such as cardiovascular disease.

The researchers looked at the similarities in chemical structure between glucose in blood and body fluids, and two other sugar called mannose and fructose. These sugars are found on the surfaces of bacteria and fungi and act as targets for receptors in our body that have evolved to detect and bind to microbial sugars to then combat the infection.

The research found that high levels of glucose outcompetes the binding of mannose and fructose to the specialized immune receptors, potentially blocking these receptors from detecting infectious bacteria and fungi. Glucose also binds in such a way that it inhibits the chemical processes that would normally then follow to combat infections. If this happens it can inhibit a range of key processes for example:

It can inhibit the function of immune system receptors called C-type lectins such as MBL (Mannose-binding lectin) which are known to bind to a sugar known as mannose that is present in the structure of infectious fungal bacterial cell walls. Unlike glucose, mannose does not exist in mammals as a free sugar in the blood.

The loss of MBL function may also predispose the body to chronic inflammatory diseases, since MBL is involved in the processing and clearance of apoptotic cells (dying cells).

A number of C-type lectins tat can be affected by raised glucose levels, including MBL, but also including immune cell surface receptors DC-SIGN and DC-SIGNR, are found in key parts of our circulation and vascular system such as plasma, monocytes, platelets and endothelial cells that line blood vessels. Inhibiting the function of these key molecules in those settings could contribute to diabetic cardiovascular and renal complications.

Warwick Medical School researcher Dr Daniel Mitchell said:

"Our findings offer a new perspective on **how high glucose can potentially affect immunity** and thus exert a negative impact on health. It also helps to emphasize the importance of good diet on preventing or controlling diseases such as diabetes. We will build on these ideas in order to consolidate the disease model and to investigate new routes to treatment and prevention."

The research will be published in the journal *Immunobiology*.

CHAPTER XII
THE HEALING POWER OF SEX

Sex is not only the most significant aspect of any successful romantic relationship but also has tremendous healing potential. In a recent study, it was revealed that individuals who indulged in regular sexual activities stayed healthier and lived longer than those who refrained from having sex!!!!!

This proves that sex not only gives you pleasure but is also a great remedy for battling an array of ailments ranging from heart disease, obesity, high blood pressure,diabetes and depression to skin disorders, stress and even cancer.

Bust Stress with Sex:

Stress can cause your blood sugar to spike. Why? Because stress causes your adrenal glands to produce the stress hormone cortisol. When you secrete cortisol, your blood sugar goes up. And when your blood sugar goes up, your pancreas produces more insulin. Too much insulin puts stress on your entire system, including inflammation of your tissues

Various modern day studies have revealed that sex is an amazing stress buster that helps lower the elevated stress levels of the body and enables you to live a happier and healthier life. Individuals having sex frequently tend to have a better response towards daily life stressors than those who abstain from it or lead a celibate lifestyle.

A big health benefit of sex is lower blood pressure and overall stress reduction, according to researchers from Scotland who reported their findings in the journal *Biological Psychology*. They studied 24 women and 22 men who kept records of their sexual activity. Then the researchers subjected them to stressful situations -- such as speaking in public and doing verbal arithmetic -- and noted their blood pressure response to stress.

Conclusion: *Since high blood pressure and stress have a big effect on diabetes it is quite clear that having more sex lowers blood sugar.*

Sex for enhancing your body's Immunity:

Good sexual health may mean better physical health. Having sex once or twice a week has been linked with higher levels of an antibody called immunoglobulin A or **IgA**, which can protect you from getting colds and other infections. Scientists at Wilkes University in Wilkes-Barre, Pa., took samples of saliva, which contain IgA, from 112 college students who reported the frequency of sex they had.

Those in the "frequent" group -- once or twice a week -- had higher levels of IgA than those in the other three groups -- who reported being abstinent, having sex less than once a week, or having it very often, three or more times weekly.

Sex can certainly boost your immune system and may even prevent you from catching cold and all types of flu.

This is because having regular sex increases the levels of immunoglobulin A, antibody. Individuals who regularly indulge in sex have higher levels of this antibody than those who rarely have sex!!!!

IT'S OFFICIAL! Sex is good for your health.

American health experts reckon sex is one of the best ways to fight off winter cold and flu bugs.

And their study suggests that people who aren't getting enough could be left feeling down in more ways than one.

Professor Carl Charnetski reported that having sex twice a week is the perfect medicine for the common cold.

"We found that individuals engaging in sex once or twice a week have substantially higher levels of antibodies than those reporting no sexual activity," he said.

His study found that having sex raised levels of the infection.

Burn Calories with Sex:

Chapter XII

Sex is considered to be one of the best forms of exercise. **As per research, about 30 minutes of great sex can lead to burning 85 calories.** A single session of sex is equivalent to around 20 laps of swimming and it also helps tone up your body muscles and enhances the flow of oxygen and blood to all body parts.

Thirty minutes of sex burns 85 calories or more. It may not sound like much, but it adds up: 42 half-hour sessions will burn 3,570 calories, more than enough to lose a pound. Doubling up, you could drop that pound in 21 hour-long sessions!!

"Sex is a great mode of exercise," says Patti Britton, PhD, a Los Angeles sexologist and president of the American Association of Sexuality Educators and Therapists. It takes work, from both a physical and psychological perspective, to do it well, she says.

Conclusion: *It is quite clear burning 3,570 calories means burning sugar!!!*

Sex Combats Depression:

Sex is one of the best known tranquilizers for treating mild cases of depression. This is because when you have sex, the happy hormones or endorphinsare released that are known to promote feelings of happiness and well being. Studies tell us that sex is 10 times more potent than Valium when it comes to treating depression and has no side effects.

Sex helps you sleep better and solves the insomnia problem:

A compound known as oxytocinis released while having sex. This is known to promote sound sleep. Sex is considered to be highly relaxing and eases the tension from every muscle of your body. It enables you to fall asleep with ease and is much safer than all those harmful sleeping pills available in the market.

The oxytocin released during orgasm also promotes sleep, according to research.

And getting enough sleep has been linked with a host of other good things, such as maintaining a healthy weight ,lower blood sugar and blood pressure. Something to think about, especially if you've been wondering why your guy can be active one minute and snoring the next.

Sex Improves Cardiovascular Health

While some older folks may worry that the efforts expended during sex could cause a stroke, that's not so, according to researchers from England. In a study published in the *Journal of Epidemiology and Community Health*, scientists found frequency of sex was not associated with stroke in the 914 men they followed for 20 years.

And the heart health benefits of sex don't end there. The researchers also found that having sex twice or more a week reduced the risk of fatal heart attack by half for the men, compared with those who had sex less than once a month.

Sex Boosts Self-Esteem

Boosting self-esteem was one of 237 reasons people have sex, collected by University of Texas researchers and published in the *Archives of Sexual Behavior.*

That finding makes sense to Gina Ogden, PhD, a sex therapist and marriage and family therapist in Cambridge, Mass., although she finds that those who already have self-esteem say they sometimes have sex to feel even better. "One of the reasons people say they have sex is to feel good about themselves," she tells WebMD. "Great sex begins with self-esteem, and it raises it. If the sex is loving, connected, and what you want, it raises it."

Sex Improves Intimacy

Having sex and orgasms increases levels of the hormone oxytocin, the so-called love hormone, which helps us bond and build trust. Researchers from the University of Pittsburgh and the University of North Carolina evaluated 59 premenopausal women before and after warm contact with their husbands and partners ending with hugs. They found that the more contact, the higher the oxytocin levels.

"Oxytocin allows us to feel the urge to nurture and to bond," Britton says.

Chapter XII

Higher oxytocin has also been linked with a feeling of generosity. So if you're feeling suddenly more generous toward your partner than usual, credit the love hormone.

Do not Miss Any Kiss

It was also found that the higher number of kisses the higher levels of the love hormone oxytocin which has an excellent positive effect on lowering blood sugar. Consistent observations on a number of diabetics at Yarmouk University Clinic who used to measure sugar level after short and long kissing sessions!!!

Sex Reduces Pain

As the hormone oxytocin surges, endorphins increase, and pain declines. So if your headache, arthritis pain, or PMS symptoms seem to improve after sex, you can thank those higher oxytocin levels.

In a study published in the *Bulletin of Experimental Biology and Medicine,* 48 volunteers who inhaled oxytocin vapor and then had their fingers pricked lowered their pain threshold by more than half.

Sex Reduces Prostate Cancer Risk

Frequent ejaculations, especially in 20-something men, may reduce the risk of prostate cancer later in life, Australian researchers reported in the *British Journal of Urology International.* When they followed men diagnosed with prostate cancer and those without, they found no association of prostate cancer with the number of sexual partners as the men reached their 30s, 40s, and 50s.

But they found men who had five or more ejaculations weekly while in their 20s reduced their risk of getting prostate cancer later by a third.

Another study, reported in the *Journal of the American Medical Association*, found that frequent ejaculations, 21 or more a month, were linked to lower prostate cancer risk in older men, as well, compared with less frequent ejaculations of four to seven monthly.

Sex Strengthens Pelvic Floor Muscles

For women, doing a few pelvic floor muscle exercises known as Kegels during sex offers a couple of benefits. You will enjoy more pleasure, and you'll also strengthen the area and help to minimize the risk of incontinence later in life.

To do a basic exercise, tighten the muscles of your pelvic floor, as if you're trying to stop the flow of urine. Count to three, then release.

Sex Improves Blood Circulation and Enhances Memory:

Mental stimulation improves brain function and actually protects against cognitive decline, as does physical exercise.
The human brain is able to continually adapt and rewire itself. Even in old age, it can grow new neurons. Severe mental decline is usually caused by disease, whereas most age-related losses in memory or motor skills simply result from inactivity and a lack of mental exercise and stimulation. In other words, use it or lose it. Walking is especially good for your brain, because it increases blood circulation and the oxygen and glucose that reach your brain running also leads to increased brain cell numbers in normal adult and elderly "senior citizen". Even sex helps to increase blood flow to the brain.

Our clinic at Yarmouk University tested the effect of sex(intercourse and kissing) on huge number of cases for different conditions and all results showed that sex has a great positive effect based on reducing stress, blood sugar,hypertension and enhancing immunity.

I myself tested its effect on my high blood pressure together with my product **PRESS OIL** which is composed of a number of essential oils and works as a natural external **vasodilator** and Iam now hypertension free since March 2008!!!My latest redings do not exceed 110/70!!!While it was 190/105 when I was diagnosed with high blood pressure!!!

For more information about this topic please visit: (ayurvediccure.com and.*webmd.com*)

Sex hormones usually act as enhancers sex drive and play a role in the reproductive system. But new studies show that sex hormones can also be used to treat diabetes.

Chapter XII

According to a new study funded by the British drug maker ProStrakan, testosterone gel therapy can fix the fundamental problems in men who suffer from diabetes type 2 (diabetes due to lifestyle).

Diabetes or insulin resistance occurs when the body does not know how to use insulin to process sugar.

The researchers found that the application of testosterone gel can reduce the problem in men with diabetes who have low testosterone levels, or in men without diabetes but with a bunch of heart risk factors called metabolic syndrome.

Testosterone gel therapy can also lower cholesterol levels and have some positive impact on sexual function.

"These findings support the treatment of testosterone in men with low testosterone and type 2 diabetes or metabolic syndrome,"explained Dr T. Hugh Jones of Barnsley Hospital in England in the journal Diabetes Care, as reported by Health24, Saturday (02/04/2011).

In this new study, researchers tested the testosterone gel ProStrakan and dummy (placebo) at 220 male middle-aged and older. Participants use the gel once a day for a year.

As a result, insulin resistance decreased by 16 percent in men who use testosterone gel. However, this testosterone gel for treatment of diabetes and the function is not a medicine to control blood sugar levels.

The researchers also found that participants were slightly increased sexual function with testosterone gel, but there was no difference in erectile dysfunction or sexual satisfaction as a whole.

The side effects were similar between the placebo gel and testosterone gel, although sometimes the testosterone gel can cause swelling around the joints and in the breast.

CHAPTER XIII
DIABETES AND ARTIFICIAL SWEETENERS

Chemical Sweeteners(Sweet Poisons)

More than 80% of diabetics use chemical sweeteners with zero calories in order to avoid any increase in blood sugar readings when they use sweetened food or drinks in the daily life. Most of those do not know about the serious fatal dangers of chemical sweeteners.

Dr. Janet Hull listed th most dangerous ones as follows (http://www.sweetpoison.com):

Information on Aspartame and Other Chemical Sweeteners:

Acesulfame K

Acesulfame Potassium (K) was approved for use by the FDA as a safe artificial sweetener in July, l988. It is a derivative of acetoacetic acid. Unfortunately, several potential problems associated with the use of acesulfame have been raised. They are based largely on animal studies since testing on humans remains limited. The findings showed the following:

Acesulfame K apparently produced lung tumors, breast tumors, rare types of tumors of other organs (such as the thymus gland), several forms of leukemia and chronic respiratory disease in several rodent studies, even when less than maximum doses were given. According to the Center for Science in the Public Interest, it was petitioned on August 29, l988 for a stay of approval by the FDA because of "significant doubt" about its safety.

Dr. H.J. Roberts, Aspartame (NutraSweet) Is It Safe?, Charles Press, page 283/84.

Aspartame

Aspartame, a dipeptide of aspartic acid and a methyl ester of phenylalanine, is approved for use in pharmaceutical products and is being used increasingly in chewable tablet and sugar-free formulations. Labels for both prescription and nonprescription products must include the phenylalanine content. The major consideration in the use of aspartame in children is in patients with autosomal recessive phenylketonuria. Although heterozygotes do not appear to have clinically significant increases in phenylalanine after ingestion of even large amounts (equivalent to 24 12-oz cans of diet beverages), homozygotes with strict dietary restrictions should avoid aspartame. Children without dietary restrictions could safely ingest 10 mg/kg/d. [37-40]. Dietary consumption of aspartame is typically less than 5 mg/kg/d[41]; young children, however, could ingest considerably more. For example, a 2-year-old child weighing 12 kg consumes 17 mg/kg from drinking one 12-oz can of diet soda and one serving of a sweetened product (eg, cereal, pudding, gelatin, or frozen dessert).

Headache is the most common adverse side effect attributed to aspartame but is seldom confirmed by single-dose double-blind challenge. Up to 11% of patients with chronic migraine headaches reported headaches triggered by aspartame; however, a double-blind challenge with three doses of 10 mg/kg given every 2 hours triggered no more headaches than did placebos in patients with vascular headaches believed to be exacerbated by aspartame. A small, double-blind 4-week trial showed an increase in frequency of headaches after ingestion of 1200 mg/d, indicating that a longer challenge period may be necessary.

In anecdotal reports, aspartame has been linked to various neuropsychiatric disorders, including panic attacks, mood changes, visual hallucinations, manic episodes, and isolated dizziness. A small, double-blind crossover study of patients with major depression revealed a higher incidence of reactions in these patients compared with non-depressed volunteers after administration of 30 mg/kg for 7 days; symptoms included headache, nervousness, dizziness, memory impairment, nausea, temper outbursts, and depression. None of these conditions has been rigorously proven to be caused by aspartame, but carefully conducted double-blind challenges may be indicated in patients with histories that suggest aspartame as a cause. Patients with underlying mitral valve prolapse or affective disorders may be at increased risk for neuropsychiatric effects; several studies have shown that individuals without psychiatric or seizure disorders do not demonstrate these effects.

Seizures have been reported via passive surveillance data collected by the FDA and in a few case reports. A recent analysis of FDA reports showed 41 cases of rechallenge with a temporal relationship to aspartame consumption. Most seizures occurred in patients who had an acceptable dietary intake, except for a 16-year-old who ingested up to 57 mg/kg of aspartame.

Saccharin

Foods containing saccharin no longer carry a label stating that the "use of this product may be hazardous to your health ...contains saccharin which has been determined to cause cancer in laboratory animals." This warning was lifted in 2001 by the American FDA as saccharin no longer has been connected to cancer in human beings.

Saccharin may be present in drugs in substantial amounts. Ingestion of the recommended daily dosage of chewable aspirin or acetaminophen tablets in a school-age child would provide approximately the same amount of saccharin contained in one can of a diet soft drink. This amount, relative to the body weight of a child younger than 9 or 10 years, ingested for prolonged periods would be considered as "heavy use," as defined in a major large-scale FDA/National Cancer Institute epidemiologic study. In this study, heavy use of artificial sweeteners was associated with a significantly increased risk for the development of bladder cancer.

Ingestion of saccharin-adulterated milk formula by infants was associated with irritability, hypertonia, insomnia, opisthotonos, and strabismus, which resolved within 36 hours after ingestion. Two anecdotal reports of an accidental overdose in an adult and a child discussed reactions of generalized edema, oliguria, and persistent albuminuria. Because of the paucity of data on the toxicity of saccharin in children, the American Medical Association has recommended limiting the intake of saccharin in young children and pregnant women.

Splenda (Sucralose)

Splenda, also known as sucralose, is an artificial sweetener, which is a chlorinated sucrose derivative. Facts about this artificial chemical are as follows:

Pre-Approval Research: Pre-approval research showed that sucralose caused shrunken thymus glands (up to 40% shrinkage) and enlarged liver and kidneys.

Recent Research:A possible problem with caecal enlargement and renal mineralization has been seen in post approval animal research.

Sucralose Breaks Down: Despite the manufacturer's misstatements, sucralose does break down into small amounts of 1,6-dichlorofructose, a chemical which has not been adequtely tested in humans. More importantly, sucralose must break down in the digestive system. If it didn't break down and react at all (as the manufacturer claims), it would not chemically-react on the tongue to provide a sweet taste. The truth is that sucralose does break down to some extent in the digestive system.

Independent, Long-Term Human Research

"100's of studies" (some of which show hazards) were clearly in adequate and do not demonstrate safety in long-term use.

Chlorinated Pesticides: The manufacturer claims that the chlorine added to sucralose is similar to the chlorine atom in the salt (NaCl) molecule. That is not the case. Sucralose may be more like ingesting tiny amounts of chlorinated pesticides, but we will never know without long-term, independent human research.

Conclusion:

While it is unlikely that sucralose is as toxic as the poisoning people are experiencing from aspartame, it is clear from the hazards seen in pre-approval research and from its chemical structure that years or decades of use may contribute to serious chronic immunological or neurological disorders.

It is very important that people who have any interest in their health stay aware from the highly toxic sweetener aspartame and other questionable sweeteners such as sucralose (Splenda), and acesulfame-k (Sunette, Sweet & Safe, Sweet One).

Aspartame Is the Most Famous and the Most Dangerous

According to (www.dorway.org) site Aspartame was not approved until 1981, in dry foods. For over eight years the FDA refused to approve it because of the seizures and brain tumors this product produced in lab

Chapter XIII ─────────────────────────

animals. The FDA continued to refuse to approve it until President Reagan took office (a friend of Searle) and fired the FDA Commissioner who wouldn't approve it. Dr. Arthur Hull Hayes was appointed as commissioner. Even then there was so much opposition to approval that a Board of Inquiry was set up. The Board said: "Do not approve aspartame". Dr. Hayes OVERRULED his own Board of Inquiry. Shortly after Commissioner Arthur Hull Hayes, Jr., approved the use of aspartame in carbonated beverages, he left for a position with G.D. Searle's Public Relations firm.

Long-Term Damage

It appears to cause slow, silent damage in those unfortunate enough to not have immediate reactions and a reason to avoid it. It may take one year, five years, 10 years, or 40 years, but it seems to cause some reversible and some irreversible changes in health over long-term use.

METHANOL (AKA WOOD ALCOHOL/POISON) (10% OF ASPARTAME)

Methanol/wood alcohol is a deadly poison. People may recall that methanol was the poison that has caused some "skid row" alcoholics to end up blind or dead. Methanol is gradually released in the small intestine when the methyl group of aspartame encounter the enzyme chymotrypsin. The absorption of methanol into the body is sped up considerably when free methanol is ingested. Free methanol is created from aspartame when it is heated to above 86 Fahrenheit (30 Centigrade). This would occur when aspartame-containing product is improperly stored or when it is heated (e.g., as part of a "food" product such as Jello).

Methanol breaks down into formic acid and formaldehyde in the body. Formaldehyde is a deadly neurotoxin. An EPA assessment of methanol states that methanol "is considered a cumulative poison due to the low rate of excretion once it is absorbed. In the body, methanol is oxidized to formaldehyde and formic acid; both of these metabolites are toxic." The recommend a limit of consumption of 7.8 mg/day. A one-liter (approx. 1 quart) aspartame-sweetened beverage contains about 56 mg of methanol. Heavy users of aspartame containing products consume as much as 250 mg of methanol daily or 32 times the EPA limit.

The most well known problems from methanol poisoning are vision problems. Formaldehyde is a known carcinogen, causes retinal damage, interferes with DNA replication, and causes birth defects. Due to the lack of a couple of key enzymes, humans are many times more sensitive to the toxic effects of methanol than animals. Therefore, tests of aspartame or methanol on animals do not accurately reflect the danger for humans. As pointed out by Dr Woodrow C. Monte, Director of the Food Science and Nutrition Laboratory at Arizona State University, "There are no human or mammalian studies to evaluate the possible mutagenic, teratogenic, or carcinogenic effects of chronic administration of methyl alcohol."

In a 1993 act that can only be described as "unconscionable", the FDA approved aspartame as an ingredient in numerous food items that would always be heated to above 86°degrees F (30°Degrees C).

Much worse, on 27 June 1996, without public notice, the FDA removed all restrictions from aspartame allowing it to be used in everything, including all heated and baked goods.

The truth about aspartame's toxicity is far different than what the NutraSweet Company would have you readers believe. In February of 1994, the U.S. Department of Health and Human Services released the listing of adverse reactions reported to the FDA (DHHS 1994). **Aspartame accounted for more than 75% of all adverse reactions reported to the FDA's Adverse Reaction Monitoring System (ARMS).** By the FDA's own admission fewer then ONE PERCENT of those who have problems with something they consume ever report it to the FDA. This balloons the almost 10,000 complaints they once had to around a million. However, the FDA has a record keeping problem (they never did respond to the certified letter from the WEBMASTER of this site... a major victim!) and they tend to discourage or even misdirect complaints, at least on aspartame. The fact remains, though, that MOST victims don't have a clue that aspartame may be the cause of their many problems!

Many reactions to aspartame were very serious including seizures and death. Those reactions included:

- Abdominal Pain
- Anxiety attacks
- Arthritis
- Asthma

Chapter XIII

- Asthmatic reactions
- Bloating, Edema (fluid retention)
- Blood Sugar Control Problems (Hypoglycemia or Hyperglycemia)
- Brain Cancer (Pre-approval studies in animals)
- Breathing difficulties
- Burning Eyes or Throat
- Burning Urination
- Can't think straight
- Chest Pains
- Chronic Cough
- Chronic Fatigue
- Confusion
- Death
- Depression
- Diarrhea
- Dizziness
- Excessive Thirst or Hunger
- Fatigue
- Feel unreal
- Flushing of face
- Hair Loss (Baldness) or Thinning of Hair
- Headaches / Migraines, Dizziness
- Hearing Loss
- Heart palpitations
- Hives (Urticaria)
- Hypertension (High Blood Pressure)

- Impotency and Sexual Problems
- Iinability to concentrate
- Infection Susceptibility
- Insomnia
- Irritability
- Itching
- Joint Pains
- Laryngitis
- "like thinking in a fog"
- Marked Personality Changes
- Memory loss
- Menstrual Problems or Changes
- Migraines and Severe Headaches (Trigger or Cause From Chronic Intake)
- Muscle spasms
- Nausea or Vomiting
- Numbness or Tingling of Extremities
- Other Allergic-Like Reactions
- Panic Attacks
- Phobias
- Poor memory
- Rapid Heart Beat
- Rashes
- Seizures and Convulsions
- Slurring of Speech
- Swallowing Pain
- Tachycardia

Chapter XIII

- Tremors
- Tinnitus
- Vertigo
- Vision Loss
- Weight gain
- Aspartame Disease Mimics Symptoms or Worsens the Following Diseases
- Fibromyalgia
- Arthritis
- Multiple Sclerosis (MS)
- Parkinson's Disease
- Lupus
- Multiple Chemical Sensitivities (MCS)
- Diabetes and Diabetic Complications
- Epilepsy
- Alzheimer's Disease
- Birth Defects
- Chronic Fatigue Syndrome
- Lymphoma
- Lyme Disease
- Attention Deficit Disorder (ADD)
- Panic Disorder
- Depression and other Psychological Disorders

How It Happens:

- Methanol, from aspartame, is released in the small intestine when the methyl group of aspartame encounters the enzyme chymotrypsin (Stegink 1984, page 143). Free methanol begins to form in liquid aspartame-containing products at temperatures

93

above 86 degrees F.. also within the human body. The methanol is then converted to formaldehyde. The formaldehyde converts to formic acid, ant sting poison. Toxic formic acid is used as an activator to strip epoxy and urethane coatings. Imagine what it does to your tissues!

- Phenylalanine and aspartic acid, 90% of aspartame, are amino acids normally used in synthesis of protoplasm when supplied by the foods we eat. But when unaccompanied by other amino acids we use [there are 20], they are neurotoxic. That is why a warning for Phenylketonurics is found on EQUAL and other aspartame products. Phenylketenurics are 2% of the population with extreme sensitivity to this chemical unless it's present in food. It gets you too, causing brain disorders and birth defects! Finally, the phenyalanine breaks down into DKP, a brain tumor agent.

- In other words: Aspartame converts to dangerous byproducts that have no natural countermeasures. A dieter's empty stomach accelerates these conversions and amplifies the damage. Components of aspartame go straight to the brain, damage that causes headaches, mental confusion, seizures and faulty balance. Lab rats and other test animals died of brain tumors.

- Despite the claims of Monsanto and bedfellows:

- 1. Methanol from alcohol and juices does not get converted to formaldehyde to any significant extent. There is very strong evidence to confirm this fact for alcoholic beverages and fairly strong evidence for juices.

- 2. Formaldehyde obtained from methanol is very toxic in *very small* doses as seen by recent research.

- 3. Aspartame causes chronic toxicity reactions/damage due to the methanol to formaldehyde and other break down products despite what is claimed otherwise by the very short, industry-funded experiments using a test substance that is chemically different and absorbed differently than what is available to the general public. "Strangely enough", almost all independent studies show that aspartame can cause health problems.

- 4. A common ploy from Monsanto is to claim that aspartame is "safe" yet a few select people may have "allergic" reactions to it.

Chapter XIII

This is typical Monsanto nonsense, of course. Their own research shows that it does not cause "allergic" reactions. It is there way of trying to minimize and hide the huge numbers of toxicity reactions and damage that people are experiencing from the long-term use of aspartame.

Summary

- Given the following points, it is definitely premature for researchers to discount the role of methanol in aspartame side effects:

- 1. The amount of methanol ingested from aspartame is unprecedented in human history. Methanol from fruit juice ingestion does not even approach the quantity of methanol ingested from aspartame, especially in persons who ingest one to three liters (or more) of diet beverages every day. Unlike methanol from aspartame, methanol from natural products is probably not absorbed or converted to its toxic metabolites in significant amounts as discussed earlier.

- 2. Lack of laboratory-detectable changes in plasma formic acid and formaldehyde levels do not preclude damage being caused by these toxic metabolites. Laboratory-detectable changes in formate levels are often not found in short exposures to methanol.

- 3. Aspartame-containing products often provide little or no nutrients which may protect against chronic methanol poisoning and are often consumed in between meals. Persons who ingest aspartame-containing products are often dieting and more likely to have nutritional deficiencies than persons who take the time to make fresh juices.

- 4. Persons with certain health conditions or on certain drugs may be much more susceptible to chronic methanol poisoning.

- 5. Chronic diseases and side effects from slow poisons often build silently over a long period of time. Many chronic diseases which seem to appear suddenly have actually been building in the body over many years.

- 6. An increasing body of research is showing that many people are highly sensitive to low doses of formaldehyde in the environment.

Environmental exposure to formaldehyde and ingestion of methanol (which converts to formaldehyde) from aspartame likely has a cumulative deleterious effect.

- 7. Formic acid has been shown to slowly accumulate in various parts of the body. Formic acid has been shown to inhibit oxygen metabolism.

- 8. The are a very large and growing number of persons are experiencing chronic health problems similar to the side effects of chronic methanol poisoning when ingesting aspartame-containing products for a significant length of time. This includes many cases of eye damage similar to the type of eye damage seen in methanol poisoning cases.

- Toxicity Effects of Aspartame Use:
  Selection of Health Effects from Short-term and/or Long-Term Use

- Note: It often takes at least sixty days without any aspartame NutraSweet to see a significant improvement. Check all labels very carefully (including vitamins and pharmaceuticals). Look for the word "aspartame" on the label and avoid it. (Also, it is a good idea to avoid "acesulfame-k" or "sunette.") Finally, avoid getting nutrition information from junk food industry PR organizations such as IFIC or organizations that accept large sums of money from the junk and chemical food industry such as the American Dietetic Association.

- If you are a user of any products with aspartame, and you have physical, visual, mental problems... take the 60-day no aspartame test. If, after two months with no aspartame your symptoms are either gone, or are much less severe, please get involved to get this neurotoxin off the market. Write a letter to the FDA, with a copy to Betty Martini (for proof of how the FDA doesn't keep proper records). Write your congressmen. Return products containing aspartame to the point of purchase... for a FULL refund. Make a big stink if they WON'T give you a full refund! Tell all your friends and family... and if they stop using aspartame and also "wake up well"... get them involved in the same way.

- Aspartame is an "approved sweetener" because of a few greedy and dishonest people who place profits above human life and well-being. With the FDA and our Congress culpable, only an INFORMED and ACTIVE public will affects its reclassification from "food additive" to TOXIC DRUG, and removed from the human food chain.

- For more information please refer to:
- http://www.dorway.com/reprtfrm.html

Neotame, the Cousin of Aspartame

Developed by Monsanto and made by NutraSweet, neotame was approved in 2002 by the Food and Drug Administration (FDA). This artificial sweetener is being used as an additive in practically anything humans consume from soft drinks, dairy products, and yogurt to frozen desserts and even chewing gum. In addition, and unlike aspartame, neotame can stand a higher temperature heat, so many food manufacturers are including it in baked goods. Neotame has become an ingredient in hundreds of food products and is often blended with other synthetic sweeteners. Most recently it has been added to the feed for some livestock being raised for human consumption

It is estimated that neotame is between 7,000 to 13,000 times sweeter than sugar, which would allow food manufacturers to use less in their products. And since the FDA does not require labels to include ingredients that contribute less than one percent of the product, in some instances neotame can be used in foods without having to be listed on the label. Neotame is also hidden under the infamous "natural flavors" category on some packaged foods.

This highly concentrated, white crystalline powder contains the same synthetic derivative of the two amino acids as aspartame - L-aspartic acid and L-phenylalanine - plus the chemical methanol, or wood alcohol. To this compound 3-dimethylbutyl has been added. NutraSweet company states that neotame is perfectly safe, yet 3-dimethylbutyl happens to be on the Environmental Protection Agency's (EPA) most hazardous chemical list.

Neotame does not have to carry the Phenylketonurics (PKU) warning on labels that include their ingredient. Phenylketonurics - or PKU - is the term used to refer to individuals that have the metabolic disorder Phenylketonuria. Those with this disorder cannot consume products that contain phenylalanine. Therefore, if products containing neotame do not include a warning label or state the ingredient is included, it could be potentially quite dangerous for these individuals.

Marketing companies claim that man-made chemical sweeteners help in the battle against obesity and in the onset of obesity-related diseases, yet statistics prove otherwise. Research has found that these artificial chemicals lead to weight gain by rapidly stimulating the release of insulin and leptin, two hormones that are directly related to satiety and fat storage.

It would seem that adding more chemicals to an already problematic chemical solution would only create more problems in the long run. At this time, long term effects on humans are unknown.

Safe and beneficial :

As recently as February, the European Food Safety Authority (EFSA) said that two recent studies linking aspartame with increased cancer rates and pre-term births *"do not give reason to reconsider previous safety assessments of aspartame or of other sweeteners currently authorised in the European Union"*

Natural Safe Sweeteners:

Dr. Janet Hull also mentioned some natural alternatives:

STEVIA

A natural sweetener, stevioside, is championed by natural-foods advocates in the United States and is used in several countries, most notably Japan. Stevioside comes from the leaves of the stevia plant (Stevia rebaudiana Bertoni), a perennial shrub native to Brazil and Paraguay. Stevia contains sweet-tasting glycosides, mainly stevioside; but also rebaudiosides A, B, C, D, and E; dulcoside A; and steviolbioside. Stevioside has a slight bitter aftertaste and provides 250 to 300 times the sweetness of sugar. It is stable to 200°C (392°F), but it is not fermentable and does not act in browning reactions.

In the 1970s, the Japanese government approved the plant for use in food. Japanese food processors use stevioside in a wide range of foods:

Chapter XIII ————————————————

pickled vegetables, dried seafood, soy sauce and miso, beverages, candy, gums, baked goods and cereals, yogurt, ice cream, and as a tabletop sweetener. In salty applications, stevioside modifies the harshness of sodium chloride. Combining it with other natural and synthetic sweeteners improves taste and functionality.

FDA considers stevia leaves and stevioside as unapproved, non-GRAS food additives. In 1992, the American Herbal Products Association (AHPA) petitioned the FDA to declare stevia as GRAS, citing historical usage and referring to numerous toxicology studies conducted in Japan and other countries. The FDA rejected AHPA's petition, contending inadequate evidence to approve the product. The agency does allow the herb to be used in dietary supplements as covered by DSHEA (Dietary Supplement Health and Education Act).

From Wikipedia:

Stevia is a genus of about 240 species of herbs and shrubs in the sunflower family (Asteraceae), native to subtropical and tropical regions from western North America to South America. The species *Stevia rebaudiana*, commonly known as **sweetleaf, sweet leaf, sugarleaf,** or simply **stevia**, is widely grown for its sweet leaves. As a sweetener and sugar substitute, stevia's taste has a slower onset and longer duration than that of sugar, although some of its extracts may have a bitter or licorice-like aftertaste at high concentrations.

With its steviol glycoside extracts having up to 300 times the sweetness of sugar, stevia has garnered attention with the rise in demand for low-carbohydrate, low-sugar food alternatives. Because stevia has a negligible effect on blood glucose, it is attractive as a natural sweetener to people on carbohydrate-controlled diets.

The availability of stevia varies from country to country. In a few countries, it has been available as a sweetener for decades or centuries; for example, stevia is widely used as a sweetener in Japan where it has been available for decades. In some countries, stevia is restricted or banned. In other countries, health concerns and political controversies have limited its availability; for example, the United States banned stevia in the early 1990s unless labeled as a dietary supplement, **but in 2008 approved rebaudioside A extract as a food additive**. Over the years, the number of countries in which stevia is available as a sweetener has been increasing.

Now there are 3 famous American, British and Canadian companies were successful in extracting efficient extracts without any bitter after taste.In Saudi Arabia stevia is sold in a form of white powder called STEVIANA.

HONEY

HONEY: For centuries, honey has been referred to as "nature's gold." After gathering the nectar from flowers and flowering plants, bees return to the hive and process the nectar as honey. The flavor of the honey reflects upon the flower. Sources commonly include buckwheat, blackberry, heather, clover, orange blossoms, wildflowers and sage. To process raw honey, remove it from its wax comb, strain or heat and filter. The downside to this process is that heating the honey destroys many of its natural enzymes and nutrients. For this reason, I highly recommend you seek out a source of raw honey, which is a much healthier alternative to the commercial pasteurized honey in most supermarkets. You can find raw honey in some health food stores or from local farmers.

Honey should be stored in a dry place. If the honey begins to crystallize, place the jar in a pot of hot water until the sugar crystals dissolve. Be careful not to make the water too hot or you risk damaging the nutrients. Honey contains the following nutrients: protein, thiamin, riboflavin, niacin, vitamin C, calcium and iron.Topical application of honey to infected wounds is an ancient remedy, and one that has been confirmed by many scientific studies.

MAPLE SYRUP AND MAPLE SUGAR

MAPLE SYRUP AND MAPLE SUGAR: To many natural food shoppers, maple syrup is the premier sweetener. Its flavor is mild and unique, yet its sweetening ability is excellent. The reason for this is that 100 percent pure Grade A maple syrup is 65 percent sucrose. Lesser grades have a slightly lower sugar content. Maple syrup is sweet stuff indeed, and when you pour it over your pancakes, remember you are getting the equivalent of half that amount of white sugar.

Maple syrup is produced in those states where nights are below freezing while the days are warm. When these temperature changes cause the sap in sugar maples, which contains 2-3 percent sucrose, to flow from the treetop down into the roots of the tree, it is tapped, collected in buckets, and then boiled down into a syrup. It takes about 40 gallons of sap to make one gallon of syrup.

TAGATOSE

It looks like sugar, tastes like sugar, cooks like sugar... well technically, it is sugar. But it's sugar with almost no calories. It's 100-percent natural - not synthesized, unlike other "sweeteners" that are chemically synthesized or derived from sugar, Tagatose is a naturally occurring sugar. And SPHERIX has discovered and patented a way to make it available for use as a food additive as well as for a variety of other uses.

It's Tagatose, the only sweetener that tastes, looks, feels, and performs like table sugar. Tagatose can supply a major need for baked goods, ice cream, chocolates, chewing gum, and other food products that can't be met by low bulk of high-intensity sweeteners. And it's safe, with over ten years of safety

It's a natural product, a chemical cousin of familiar sugars such as sucrose, fructose, dextrose and lactose. Tagatose, like table sugar, is a white crystal; it is 90 percent as sweet as ordinary sugar, but has one-third the calories.

Diabetics can eat foods sweetened with tagatose without getting the unhealthful changes in their blood glucose levels that are caused by eating sugar.

ERYTHRITOL

Erythritol is a natural sugar alcohol (a type of sugar substitute) which has been approved for use in the United States and throughout much of the world. It is 70% as sweet as table sugar and excellent-tasting, yet it is virtually non-caloric, does not affect blood sugar, does not cause tooth decay, and is absorbed by the body, therefore unlikely to cause gastric side effects unlike other sugar alcohols. Under U.S. FDA labeling requirements, it has a caloric value of 0.2 calories per gram (95% less than sugar and other carbohydrates), but other countries such as Japan label it at 0 calories.

LO HAN KUO

Lo Han Kuo is the fruit of Momordica grosvenori, a plant cultivated in the mountains of southern China. Mogrosides, which are water extracted from the Lo Han fruit, offer a pleasant, sweet taste without elevating blood sugar. Lo Han Kuo Mogrosides are up to 250x sweeter than sugar.

XYLITOL

Xylitol, a naturally occurring polyol, is sweet with a distinct cooling sensation in the mouth. Xylitol is metabolized differently from a conventional sugar and does not cause or contribute to tooth decay. Xylitol is as sweet as sugar, having 40% less calories.

CHAPTER IXV

DIABETES AND CAMEL MILK

Unlike all types of milks, camel milk posseses unique health and medicinal properties that makes it on the top of all existing products.

Ingredients

Camel milk is rich on non-saturated fatty acids, iron, Vitamins B and C. Especially in Africa and Asia it is greatly valued for its health benefits. It is a valuable alternative for those persons suffering from allergy against cow milk. Camel milk also contains lactose but is an non-allergic organic product.

Medicinal Uses of Camel Milk

Prophet Muhammad (Peace Be Upon Him) described camel milk and its urine for liver cirrhosis in one of narrations in AL-BUKHARI BOOK:

Narrated by Anas: ((Some people from the tribe of 'Ukl came to the Prophet and embraced Islam. The climate of Medina did not suit them, so the Prophet ordered them to go to the (herd of milch) camels of charity and to drink, their milk and urine (as a medicine). They did so, and after they had recovered from their liver ailment became healthy)).

A number of our patients used this prescription for liver cirrhosis and all of them were cured.After many successful cases we capsulated dried camel milk with other herbs under the name : **CAMEL TECH.**

After that our patients used camel milk with urine or without urine mixed with black seed or cinnamon and it did give excellent results in:

- Treatment to decrease or remove the ulceration of the human skin, especially those who are injured.
- Treatment of burns (and sunburn)
- Treatment for the reduction of noticeable scarring
- Treatment to prevent skin and diaper rashes on babies. Actually, rashes occur also between the legs of older persons and this is

easily removed by rubbing camel milk creams on the affected areas. Two additions with gentle rubbing remove the rash within two days.

• Treatment for joint and muscle pains

When used as a massage cream for these areas, the benefits are observed within minutes and no messy traces is left after its use as it all penetrates into the skin.

• Treatment for hemorrhoids (in Arabic "basour") either used alone with a piece of cotton or mixed with Vaseline and olive oil.

• Treatment for the stretch marks of pregnant women inside DR.MANSOUR'S Glow Tech Dead Sea Cream

• Treatment for easing the pain of varicose veins

• Treatment for soft bleeding gums and cleaning teeth.

• Treatment of Daibetic Gangrene.

A few drops of camel milk when added to tooth paste or alone on a tooth brush and rubbed on the teeth gives hardening, cleaning and removal of pain, as well as removal of plaque of accumulated bacteria and leftover food materials between the teeth. It also causes whitening of the teeth.

• Massage cream. This general usage has proven its superiority to other massage products.

• As an aftershave cream which leaves no trace of it on the skin but makes it soft.

• As a pre-shave natural liquid cream which makes it easy to shave.

• As a softener for dry skin treatment to the hands. This is almost instantly observed when rubbing a few drops into the hands.

• As a treatment to hair loss on the face and skin. When a few drops are used daily, the results of removing what they call "talabinah" in Arabic are remarkable, as tested on many individuals locally.

• As a night cream for ladies and even men to prevent wrinkles and minimize their formation.

Chapter IVX

- For young ladies as a cream treatment to the rash forming after hair removal from ladies legs and under the arms

- As an excellent treatment to the hair fall when added to Prof.Mansour's SMART Shampoo.

- As a preventer and inhibitor of fungus and bacterial infection in the urinary tract of ladies, utilizing camel milk in spray form.

- As a preventer for hair loss before the death of hair follicles – but not necessarily restoration. camel milk /urine keep the hair appearance fresh from aging and harsh shampoos.

- As an improver added to any creams, conditioners and shampoos as is now used by the cosmetic industry by using only a small percent of the camel milk

- As an effective treatment to prevent athletes foot, cold feet and dry feet

- Last but not least, as a treatment to prevent bedsores for those who have to stay in bed due to some injury, as occurring often in Palestine .

Cosmetic Uses of Camel Milk

Our patients also used it :

1-As a powerful massage milk and pain killer for joints,muscles,neck,back,knee & foot.

2-For treating baby rash- a 100% sure remedy.

3-For treating burns and sun-burns.

4-For preventing urinary tract infection in females.

5-For preventing fungus.

6-For treating hemmrohids and varicose veins.

7-For cellulite and fat deposits on stomach ,legs.

8-For Eczema and Psoriasis.

9-For preventing wrinkles.

10-For softening skin

In Internal Medicinal Uses:

1-For preventing cough when mixed with honey.

2-For preventing smoker's cough

3-For relieving contispation.

4-For treating stomach ulcer

5-For preventing acid reflux

6-For weight loss

7-For all types of Cancer

8-For ulcerative colitis

9-For Diabetes I & II

10-The only hope for liver cirrhosis

11-For Lupus(SLE)

12-For Rheumatoid Arthtritis

13- For Energy & Vitality .

14-For Sexual Energy

15- For Heart Problems.

16-For Infertility

17-For Eye Disorders.

18-For Crohn's Disease

19-For all Immune & Auto-Immune Diseases.

20- For Stress & Hypertension.

Camel Milk May Be Answer to Diabetes?

By Dr. R.P.Agrawal, International Journal of Diabetes

It has been scientifically proven that gulping down camel milk daily would cut 60 to 70 per cent of insulin in Type I diabetics.

According to the research conducted at the Diabetes Care and Research Centre, SP Medical College Bikaner, a litre of camel milk contains about 52 units of insulin.

Chapter IVX

"These units in camel milk are not neutralized by the acidic juices in the stomach, unlike other forms of orally administered insulin," said Mr RP Agrawal, director, Diabetes Care and Research Centre, Bikaner.

It has been scientifically proven that gulping down camel milk daily would cut 60 to 70 percent of insulin in Type I diabetics.

The research on the project had begun with the Raica community as the base model. An initial survey revealed zero prevalence among the Raicas in Jaisalmer and Jodhpur, while the rest of the tribe members in the same region who do not like camel milk but have similar lifestyles, had five to six per cent prevalence. Camel milk was successfully tested on albino rats clinically induced with diabetes. Later, similar tests were conducted on more than 50 individuals with Type I and Type II diabetes for more than two years, resulting in a drastic fall in their blood sugar levels.

"A Type I diabetic who needs 20 units of insulin can bring this down to six to seven units with regular intake of camel milk," he said. Both camel milk and this batch of researchers from Bikaner are yet to get their due in their own diabetes-infested country. But they have featured in many international journals and research publications and even been recommended by the American Diabetes Association.

The Indian Council of Medical Research (ICMR) recently recognized this unique discovery which could provide an effective relief to scores of diabetics in the country.

"Sadly, most of the people in our country are unaware of the fact. But, we are in correspondence with medical universities and research institutes in the USA," Dr Agrawal said.

Scientists are attributing this trait of camel milk to a unique phytonutrient (derived from plants) present in the camels' daily diet. But they are yet to isolate this blood sugar fighting agent. Research is on. Camel milk is also high on minerals and low on cholesterol content, compared to cow's milk.

From many recent studies there is clear evidence that regular camel milk consumption contributes to an optimum diabetes management.

CHAPTER XV
DIABETES AND VITAMIN D

Low Vitamin D Linked to Poor Diabetes Control
Study Finds Vitamin D Deficiency Common in People With Diabetes

Kathleen Doheny from WebMed Health wrote:

June 21, 2010 -- Vitamin D deficiency, long suspected to be a risk factor for glucose intolerance, is commonly found in people with poor diabetes control, according to a new study.

"Our study could not show cause and effect," says Esther Krug, MD, an endocrinologist at Sinai Hospital of Baltimore and assistant professor of medicine at Johns Hopkins University School of Medicine, Baltimore, who presented the findings at ENDO 2010, the annual meeting of The Endocrine Society, in San Diego.

But she did find that vitamin D deficiency was common in her study, with more than 91% of participants deficient. As the deficiency worsened, so did diabetes control. Only eight of the 124 participants took vitamin D supplements, she found.

Mathieu C. et al from Catholic University of Leuven, Belgium summarized their new study as follows:

Vitamin D deficiency predisposes individuals to type 1 and type 2 diabetes, and receptors for its activated form-1alpha,25-dihydroxyvitamin D3-have been identified in both beta cells and immune cells. Vitamin D deficiency has been shown to impair insulin synthesis and secretion in humans and in animal models of diabetes, suggesting a role in the development of type 2 diabetes. Furthermore, epidemiological studies suggest a link between vitamin D deficiency in early life and the later onset of type 1 diabetes. In some populations, type 1 diabetes is associated with certain polymorphisms within the vitamin D receptor gene. In studies in non-obese diabetic mice, pharmacological doses of 1alpha,25-dihydroxyvitamin D3, or its structural analogues, have been shown to delay the onset of diabetes, mainly through immune modulation. Vitamin D deficiency may, therefore, be involved in the pathogenesis of both forms of diabetes, and a better understanding of the mechanisms involved could lead to the development of preventive strategies.

Dr. Mansour

New research indicates a good dose of Vitamin D can help protect you against diabetes. Researchers have found that low blood levels of Vitamin D interfere with the proper function of insulin-producing cells, Beta cells.. Low Vitamin D levels also result in an increase in the risk of insulin resistance, even in otherwise healthy individuals. So sunshine is necessary for you to increase your own Vitamin D levels

Vitamin D-fortified yogurt improves blood sugar control in diabetics

Dr. John Briffa wrote on 03/20/2011 :

Previously I have covered some of the evidence linking vitamin D with positive health outcomes, including a reduced risk of cardiovascular disease and several forms of cancer.

Vitamin D has also been linked with diabetes, in that some studies have found those with higher levels of vitamin D to be a reduced risk of this condition. There has also been a little evidence that supplementation with vitamin D and/or calcium may have some benefit in terms of blood sugar control. There's a hint, therefore, that higher intakes of these nutrients might reduce the risk of type-2 diabetes.

Recently, a study was published which assessed the impact of giving nutrient fortified yogurt to individuals with type-2 diabetes. Ninety individuals were treated with one of the following each day:

1. 500 mls of plain yogurt

2. 500 mls of plain yogurt containing 1000 IU of vitamin D3 and 300 mg of calcium

3. 500 mls plain yogurt containing 1000 IU of vitamin D3 and 500 mg of calcium

A range of body and biochemical measurements were assessed at the beginning and end of the study

At the beginning of the study, about three-quarters of the study participants were deemed to be 'insufficient' in vitamin D (vitamin D3 level 27.5 – >50.0 nmol/l = 11.0-20.0 ng/ml). About 40 per cent were deemed to have severe deficiency (<27.5 nmol/l = 11.0 ng/ml).

Chapter XV

At the end of the study, vitamin D levels had risen significantly in groups 2. and 3. Relative rise was about 75 per cent in both groups, which corresponded to an absolute rise of 30-35 nmol/l (12.0-14.0 ng/ml).

Those in groups 2. and 3. saw <u>significant</u> reductions in:

- Weight
- Body mass index
- Waist circumference
- Fasting blood sugar (glucose) level
- HbA1c level (gives a guide to blood sugar levels over the preceding 2-3 months)

As well as improvement in markers of insulin sensitivity (to an extent comparable to treatment with the diabetes drug metformin).

The authors of this study conclude that vitamin D fortified yogurt (with or without additional calcium) helped blood sugar control in type-2 diabetics probably through direct effects on insulin sensitivity and indirectly also through improvements in weight.

One interest thing to note about this study was just how effective vitamin D-supplemented yogurt was in raising vitamin D levels. Vitamin D is fat-soluble, and it's just possible, I suppose, that the fat in the yogurt enhanced the absorption and 'bioavailability' of the vitamin D.

VITAMIN D DOSAGE: A minimum of 10,000 I.U. of Vitamin D daily. This is absolutely required in order for your body to absorb the coral calcium.

CHAPTER XVI
DIABETES AND TESTOSTERONE

Using Testosterone to Reverse Type 2 Diabetes in Men

Treating Diabetes in Men by Lichten Approach

By Edward Lichten, MD :

Type 2 diabetes is a chronic and life-shortening disease characterized by insulin resistance from an overabundance of stored glycogen. Insulin resistance causes the abnormal laboratory findings of hyperglycemia (high blood sugar), hyperinsulinemia and elevated glycosylated hemoglobin (HbA1c). The majority of individuals with heart disease, renal disease necessitating dialysis, retinopathy and amputation suffer from diabetes. A reduction in insulin resistance, serum glucose, fasting insulin and HbA1c has been observed in men treated with injectible testosterone.

An estimated 20 million Americans have diabetes. More than 90% have type 2 diabetes. For these people, an overproduction of insulin cannot control elevated blood glucose. By contrast, people with type 1 diabetes produce little or no insulin (hypoinsulinemia) due to destruction of their islet cells. The incidence of diabetes has increased 6 fold since 1958.

At present there is no cure for diabetes , and there have been no medical breakthroughs since Banting and Best discovered insulin in 1922. [once diabetes has been diagnosed]medical treatment with oral hypoglycemic agents and insulin is offered to patients to "lower" their serum glucose.

This approach, however, fails to address the true physiology of type 2 diabetes. Hollenbeck and Reaven documented a stepwise increase in insulin response within the standard glucose tolerance test in which the lowest quartile had insulin of less then 8 uU/ml and a one hour insulin above 70 (Journal of Clinical Endocrine Metabolism, 1987). Since insulin is released in response to elevated serum glucose, hyperinsulinemia and an increased insulin response to glucose are the first measureable steps in the diagnosis of insulin resistance.

It is proposed that the underlying physiology of insulin resistance is a defect in the utilization of glycogen within the cell. Since 80% of glucose is stored in the muscle and only 20% is stored in the liver, this defect primarily affects glycogen utilization within the muscle, preventing the muscle from using glycogen stores. Increasing glycogen stores inhibits the transportation of glucose across the cell membrane for storage. This resistance to glucose entering the cells results in an elevated serum glucose (hyperglycemia), which causes an increased release of insulin (hyperinsulinemia).

Lowering blood glucose with oral agents or forcing more glucose into the cell with increasing levels of insulin does not address the underlying physiologic problem of resistance. These disease processes continue as increasing glycogen deposits magnify the problems of obesity, which in turn, increases insulin resistance.

UNDERSTANDING INSULIN

For 400 million years, animals have produced insulin to store glucose as glycogen for later energy utilization. In small doses, insulin is an anabolic steroid that optimizes lean body mass and energy utilization. In excess, however, insulin impairs cyclic-AMP, inhibits release of anabolic steroids, increases catabolic processes and decreases the energy available to the organism. Levels less then 8 mIU/ml are optimal to maintaining good health.

Endocrinologists successfully treat diseases of hormone insuffieciency-hypothyroidism,hypoadrenalism, hypogonadism, somatotrophin dificiency (low growth hormone) - by supplementing with hormones, and diseases of excess hormonal production - hyperthyroidism, hypercortisolism and somatrophin excess (gigantism) by destroying or blocking hormones. This, treating hyperinsulinism with more insulin is simply illogical.

TESTOSTERONE TREATMENT

Moller and other European clinicians used testosterone to treat people with severe diabetes in the 1960's and 1970's . In 1996, we offered a few of our male patients with severe diabetes a testosterone treatment protocol.

Dr. Lichten then lists case histories of 4 severe diabetics who had tremendous improvements using testosterone to improve their diabetes.

Chapter XVI ─────────────────────

These patients also had dramatic weight loss and improved sexual function.

SEX HORMONE BINDING GLOBULIN

Sex hormone binding globulin (SHBG) is the ligand that binds testosterone, dihydrotestosterone and estradiol to the cell wall. Without SHBG , no gonadal hormone can enter the cell, penetrate the nucleus and generate release of m-RNA to cause gene expression. men have much less SHBG then women because men need to "turn on" testosterone receptors to remain male. SHBG has been shown to be an estrogen amplifier (Clinical Endocrinology 1972). Elevated SHBG and estradiol are found in men with central obesity, gynocomastia and type 2 diabetes.

Normal men have more free testosterone then free estradiol only when there is adequate testosterone and SHBG less than 15 pmol/L (Clinical Endocrinology 1972). An increase in SHBG preferentially binds testosterone over estradiol, shifting the ratio to greater free estradiol over testosterone, a state that is not conducive to normal male function.

Parenteral testosterone (injections and pellets) can help reverse the shift to estradiol dominance by increasing testosterone levels and lowering SHBG.

PREVIOUS MEDICAL RESEARCH

Our observations during testosterone replacement are consistent with previous medical publications. Haffner noted that low levels of testosterone are found in diabetic men, stating that "The absence of testosterone is..followed by insulin resistence that is localized to diminished insulin-sensitive glycogen synthase activity and is totally reversible by testosterone substitution" (American Journal of Epidemiology 1996). Tibblin reiterated this finding "...data from intervention studies suggest that the low secretion of testosterone might be a primary event in the pathogenesis of insulin resistance, because the replacement of testosterone to normal values reduces insulin resistance " (Diabetes 1996).

Our research into the function of sex hormone binding globulin has taken us one step further toward understanding the interactions of testosterone and insulin homeostasis in the male.

In short by adding testosterone it lowers SHBG. Lowering SHBG lowers the estrogen/testosterone ratio and also lowers insulin. Lowering insulin reduces angina, heart disease and obesity]

FUTURE APPLICATIONS

In 1987, Reaven coined the term syndrome X as a synonym for hyperinsulinemia (Diabetes 1988). he concluded the following disease states within syndrome X, all of which have the underlying physiology of hyperinsulinemia:

* Impaired glucose tolerance and type 2 diabetes

* Obesity

* Hypertension

* Dyslipidemia

* Heart disease

Kaplan also has observed that hyperinsulinemia precedes these disease states (Archives of Internal Medicine 1989). Depres notes that the risk of ischemic heart disease in men is 5.5 times higher with elevated insulin levels (New England Journal of Medicine 1996), and Zmuda has observed that a decrease in endogenous testosterone is associated with an increase in triglycerides and decrease in HDL cholesterol (American Journal of Epidemiology 1997).

We postulate that type 2 diabetes in men is usually a state of relative hypogonadism as well as hyperinsulinemia and that testosterone is the appropriate gender specific treatment. Birkeland observes "... a direct correlation between sensitivity to insulin and SHBG in men with type 2 diabetes " (Journal of Clinical Endocrine Metabolism 1993). Haffner also supports the concept of testosterone supplementation noting that "increased testosterone and DHEAS-SO4... is associated with lower insulin in men" and that adding testosterone to centrally obese middle aged men has improved insulin sensitivity (Hormone Research 1996 and Metabolic Clinical Experiment 1994).

Based on these findings some of our male patients started to take our natural dietary supplement VITA-X which includes a number of herbs which boost production of testosterone such as: Mucuna Pruriens,Tongkat Ali, Horny Goat Weed, Tribulis Terrestris, Saw Palmetto and L-Arginine. All of patients found improvement in their sugar level and sexual functions.

CHAPTER XVII

DIABETES AND HEALING EFFECTS OF BIOMAGNETS , ACUPUNCTURE &ULTRASOUND

While there is no definitive cure for diabetes, the search for comprehensive treatments for the condition remains constant. Lately, alternative treatments are being preferred in place of traditional medication generally administered for diabetes. Magnetic therapy is one such alternative treatment which may help cure diabetes.

Although not scientifically proven and controversial, theories suggest biomagnets alone do not heal but rather stimulate the body to heal naturally. Magnetic therapy theory includes:

-Restoration of cellular magnetic balance

-Migration of calcium ions is accelerated to help heal bones and nerve tissues

-Circulation is enhanced since biomagnets are attracted to the iron in blood and this increase in blood flow helps healing.

-Biomagnets have a positive effect on the pH balance of cells (It was observed blood samples with a pH tendency to acidity and how after being treated by Dr. Goiz magnetic therapy the acidity in those blood samples to

tally disappeared. Just with the magnets and in 15 minutes)

-Hormone production is influenced by biomagnet use

While the effectiveness of magnets to treat diabetes is still under research, there are both- the supporters as well as the critics of the method. The simple theory behind its effectiveness lies in the power of the magnets to heat and move. This quality may help expand blood vessels, thereby improving the blood flow. What's more, magnetic therapy is non evasive and can be used to cure diabetes safely.

Things to remember before opting for magnetic therapy

* Educate yourself about how a magnet may be beneficial to your health and especially to your diabetic condition. Most diabetics experience poor blood circulation in hands and feet characterized by numbness or needle like sensation. Magnets can help the condition by improving the blood flow to the legs and thereby, relieving the swelling.

* The pancreas gland may be stimulated with the help of two magnets placed on the back, above the location of the navel. They should be relatively strong and you should use them twice a day for fifteen minutes every time. They can help increase the insulin quantity produced by the body.

* Drinking 3-4 cups of magnetized water each day can boost the effectiveness of the magnets you place on your back. The water will also increase your blood flow while simultaneously reducing inflammation. Magnetized water may also help in regulating hormones along with blood sugar levels.

* Magnetic insoles for shoes can also help control diabetes. They are widely available and provide great comfort to diabetic patients suffering from peripheral neuropathy.

* Try walking to do away with any pain. The insole magnet will improve the blood circulation in your feet. Some may even increase the working of natural painkillers present in the body as well as of endorphins.

* Water wand: magnetism absorbed in the blood stream can both reduce inflammation and improve blood circulation. It is also said to help in the detoxification process of the body. 4-6 glasses of magnetized water a day can lower blood sugar levels significantly. Remember to check the levels though.

While magnetic therapy is not a permanent cure, it does has its impact on the mechanism of the peripheral nerves. Additional research is being carried out to check whether it promotes nerve cell regeneration as well or not.

Therefore, while further studies need to be conducted to determine the exact effectiveness of magnetic therapy for diabetes; diabetics definitely have a ray of hope.

Magnetic Diabetes Belt

The manufacturers of the magnetic belt claim that by placing magnetic side of the belt to pancreas it controls diabetes by stimulating pancreas!!!

ACUPUNCTURE THERAPY

Treating Diabetes with Acupuncture and Chinese Medicine

In treating diabetes, Oriental medicine offers a way to address each patient individually to eliminate the symptoms associated with diabetes and reduce the need for insulin. The practitioner may choose to use a variety of techniques during treatment including acupuncture, Chinese herbal medicine, bodywork, lifestyle/dietary recommendations and energetic exercises. The treatment for diabetes will focus on regulating the circulation of blood and balancing the organ systems to improve pancreatic function and address internal heat and the depletion of fluids. A number of studies were performed to prove the positive effect of acupuncture on diabetes and its complications. In Islamic culture we can find what is called "HIJAMA" which is a type of acupuncture

Used by Prophet Muhammad (Peace Be Upon Him) in the 6th Century to treat a number of diseases by getting rid of dirty blood every 6 months.

ULTRASOUND THERAPY

Ultrasound therapy for recalcitrant diabetic foot ulcers: results of a randomized, double-blind, controlled, multicenter study.

By: Ennis WJ, Foremann P, Mozen N, Massey J, Conner-Kerr T, Meneses P.

Wound Treatment Program, Advocate Christ Medical Center, 4440 West 95th Street, Oak Lawn, IL 60453, USA. (Ostomy Wound Manage. 2005 Sep;51(9):14).

An estimated 15% of patients with diabetes will develop a foot ulcer sometime in their life, making them 30 to 40 times more likely to undergo amputation due to a non-healing foot ulcer than the non-diabetic population. To determine the safety and efficacy of a new, non-contact, kilohertz ultrasound therapy for the healing of recalcitrant diabetic foot ulcers - as well as to evaluate the impact on total closure and quantitative bacterial cultures and the effect on healing of various levels of

119

sharp/surgical debridement - a randomized, double-blinded, sham-controlled, multicenter study was conducted in hospital-based and private wound care clinics. Patients (55 met criteria for efficacy analysis) received standard of care, which included products that provide a moist environment, off loading diabetic shoes and socks, debridement, wound evaluation, and measurement. The "therapy" was either active 40 KHz ultrasound delivered by a saline mist or a "sham device" which delivered a saline mist without the use of ultrasound. After 12 weeks of care, the proportion of wounds healed (defined as complete epithelialization without drainage) in the active ultrasound therapy device group was significantly higher than that in the sham control group (40.7% versus 14.3%, P = 0.0366, Fisher's exact test). The ultrasound treatment was easy to use and no difference in the number and type of adverse events between the two treatment groups was noted. Of interest, wounds were debrided at baseline followed by a quantitative culture biopsy. The results of these cultures demonstrated a significant bioburden (greater than $10(5)$) in the majority of cases, despite a lack of clinical signs of infection. Compared to control, this therapeutic modality was found to increase the healing rate of recalcitrant, diabetic foot ulcers.

Ultrasound therapy for Diabetes

A number of our diabetics of both types used a HIFU (High Intensity Focused Ultrasound)machine on their pancreas for 15 minutes and they were surprised by the blood glucose readings reduction.Dr.B.Khasawneh said it is early to conclude the effect of ultrasound external effect on diabetes.It needs a double blind extensive clinical trials.

CHAPTER XVIII
DIABETES AROMATHERAPY & REFLEXOLOGY

Aromatherapy is an old well-known method of healing naturally by using essential oils of plants.Aromatherapy puts to use the immense benefits of the natural extracts of medicinal plants. These natural extracts which are known as essential oils have medicinal properties to treat various disorders with the aroma of the oils. The essential oils are extracts from a plant's flowers, leaves, stalks, bark, rind, or roots.

Practitioners of aromatherapy believe that fragrances in the oils stimulate nerves in the nose and interact with the body's hormones and enzymes to cause changes in blood pressure, pulse, and other functions of the body.

It is important to note that essential oils are either applied to skin, inhaled or sprayed in the air and an intake of essential oil is considered to have some harmful effects if amounts of oils exceed certain limits.

Though various studies prove that aromatherapy cannot cure diabetes. It can surely reduce the alarming side effects of diabetes such as numbness and painful nerve disorder and also reduce infections.

Healing Power of Diabetes Massage with Essential Oils

Massage with Essential Oils improves circulation. This improved flow delivers more oxygen and nutrition. It even helps medication work better! At the same time, massage helps rid the body of toxins.

Moreover massage is the quickest way to improve the health of someone with diabetes since it reduces stress and depression if they are used on proper parts of the body; and the patients who used our aromatherapy oil mix ; **RELAX U PERFUME** reported excellent findings; they rid of numbness in arms, legs, fingers or foot. They also got rid of stress when they used it with gentle massage on nose moving up on eyebrows and forehead.

A foot bath is ideal for diabetes. Essential oils such as Rosemary, Geranium, Ginger, Cypress, Lavender, Juniper or Hyssop can be added to warm water for a foot bath.

• Massaging the feet, legs, hands and arms with any of these aromatherapy oils may improve blood circulation.

• Some essential oils, used by professionals in the correct measure for a session of massage therapy may prove beneficial to diabetics. Essential oils used by therapists for massage include: Rosemary, Lemon ,Juniper and Geranium oils with vegetable oil base.

To get more benefits of aromatherapy with essential oils we mixed number of them with some herbal extracts and a honey base cream and made a FOOT CARE CREAM which is easier to be used as a massage cream on foot and leg than pure essential oils. Moreover it heals foot cracks , moistens the skin and fights foot ulcer ,wounds and amputation.

Diabetes Sugar Lowering Essential Oils

Aromatherapy practitioners happen to be prescribing numerous essential oils that have diabetes sugar levels lowering qualities. Cypress, Dill, Fennel, Coriander and Cinnamon aromatherapy essential oils are a few of them.These essential oils also help unblock the blocked receptor areas which cause cells to become resistant against the influences of insulin.

• There is some evidence indicating therapeutic benefits by oral intake of herbs such as Asian ginseng , Fenugreek , and Aloe Vera known to improve glucose tolerance which is beneficial for diabetics.

• Many essential oils have been prescribed by therapists as having a blood sugar lowering effect .Dill, coriander, and fennel essential are some of them.

The essential oils Cypress, Geranium, Rosemary and Lemon are excellent for normalizing the circulatory system. One drop of Lemon essential oil may be dissolved in each glass of water .This drink many times a day will help maintaining healthy arteries and veins.

We filled 300ml of essential oils inside capsules and hundreds of TYPE I & II diabetics took 2 capsules daily and they were amazed by their new low sugar levels and some them left insulin under their doctors supervision!!!

Diabetes and Reflexology

The Reflexology Association of Canada defines it as "A natural healing art, based on the principle that there are reflexes in the feet and

Chapter XVIII ──────────────

hands which correspond to every part of the body." By stimulating and applying pressure to the feet or hands, you are increasing circulation and promoting specific bodily and muscular functions. Kevin Kunz, one of the pioneers of reflexology, puts it best -- "Imagine stepping on a tack. Your whole body reacts because of something perceived by the foot. Reflexology with a full range of pressure sensors, utilizes the same body system of fight or flight to relax the body."

The 1996 China Reflexology Symposium Report has found **foot reflexology** to be **93.63% effective in treating 63 disorders**. After an analysis of 8,096 clinical cases, Dr. Wang Liang reported that reflexology was significantly effective (the cure) in 48.68% of all the cases, and an effective/improved treatment in 44.95% of the cases.

Another study, in Britain, had fifteen women receive half-hour reflexology sessions for eight weeks. The findings included noticable physical and emotional improvements, increased self-esteem and confidence, an ability to stay motivated and be heard and taken seriously, and an improvement in concentration.

Double blind study with a control group. 22 cases with non-insulin dependent diabetes split into two groups. The patients of both groups had taken hypoglycemic agents for a long time. Foot reflexotherapy was applied once a day for thirty days.

Results: Indexes of the scores of senility, thrombocyte aggregation rates (TAR), the length and wet weights of thrombosis in vitro, and the serum oxidative lipids were measured to judge curative effect. The foot reflexotherapy group showed a "marked improvement" with a 66.7% "effective rate" in the measured indices. It is termed a "satisfactory curative effect." The non-foot reflexolotherapy showed no significant change 20% effective rate.

The blood flow rate was tested by color Doppler ultrasonic examination before and after foot reflexotherapy for a treatment group of 20 individuals with Type II diabetes and a control group of 15 individuals with no Type II diabetes and no diseases affecting arterial blood flow in the lower limbs. Results: There were significant differences in the blood flow rate to the feet of Type II diabetes individuals before and after application of technique. The blood flow rate of diabetic individuals was lower than those in the control group. Ying,

Ma, "Clinical Observation on Influence upon Arterial Blood Flow in the Lower Limbs of 20 Cases with Type II Diabetes Mellitus Treated by Foot Reflexology," 1998 China Reflexology Symposium Report, China Reflexology Association, Beijing, pp. 97 – 99

AROMA DIA CREAM

We formulated a cream based on some essential oils and herbal extracts called DIA CREAM which was used by diabetics of both types on **foot** and on **navel** (clinically known as the **umbilicus**, also known as the **belly button**).Some diabetics informed us that his/her blood sugar was reduced up to 100 units with one single application on either foot or **umbilicus** and the results were better when it was used on umblicus!! A double blind study is needed to be performed in order to confirm our findings.

CHAPTER IXV
DIABETES HEALING
FOODS,HERBS,VITAMINS,MINERALS AND SUPPLEMENTS

If you are serious to revesrse diabetes and live healthy life without complications here is a list of the most important foods ,herbs, vitamins ,minerals that every diabetic needs to know:

HERBS FOR DIABETES

We list here the most important and famous anti-diabetic and hypoglycemic herbs known to scientists:

Alfalfa : The name is derived from Arabic word and means "father of all foods".Is is rich in vitamins including A,D,E and K, minerals, chlorophyll and protein. It is diuretic, and it is useful for ulcer ,arthritis ,edema, and it helps prevent heart attack ,strokes and studies at the University of California at Davis found that Alfalfa extract with Manganese did improve the condition of diabetics who failed to respond to insulin.

Aloe Vera: The inner portions of the Aloe vera leaves contain a gel. This gel has water-soluble fiber that may help to reduce the absorption of carbohydrates by the intestines. In clinical trials using juice made from Aloe gel, people with type 2 diabetes reported decreased fasting blood glucose and HbA1c levels. No adverse effects were seen in these trials.

Asian Ginseng: Asian ginseng is commonly used in traditional Chinese medicine to treat diabetes. It has been shown to enhance the release of insulin from the pancreas and to increase the number of insulin receptors. It also has a direct blood sugar-lowering effect.Besides reducing fasting blood sugar levels and body weight, can elevate mood and improve psycho- physiological performance.

Asparagus Racemosus Root: has previously been reported to reduce blood glucose in rats and rabbits. In the present study, the effects of the extract and five partition fractions of the root of A.Racemosus were evaluated on insulin secretion together with exploration of their mechanisms of action. Future work assessing the use of this plant as a source of active components may provide new opportunities for diabetes therapy.

Banaba Leaf :Banaba grows in the Philippines, India, Malaysia and Australia. Banaba possesses the powerful compound corosolic acid and tannins, that lends itself to the treatment of diabetes. These ingredients are thought to stimulate glucose uptake and have insulin-like activity. The latter activity is thought to be secondary to activation of the insulin receptor tyrosine kinase or the inhibition of tyrosine phosphatase. It is a natural plant insulin, can be taken orally.

Bilberry: Bilberry leaves have traditionally been used to control blood sugar levels in people with diabetes. Bilberry has also been suggested as a treatment for retinopathy (damage to the retina) because anthocyanosides appear to help protect the retina. Bilberry has also been suggested as treatment to prevent cataracts.

Bitter Melon Fruit (Karela): Also known as bitter gourd, bitter cucumber, karela, and charantin; is a tropical vegetable widely cultivated in Asia, East Africa and South America, and has been used extensively in folk medicine as a remedy for diabetes. Studies suggested that Asian Bitter Melon may lower blood glucose concentrations. Several compounds have been isolated from bitter melon that are believed to be responsible for its blood-sugar-lowering properties. These include charantin and an insulin-like protein referred to as polypeptide-P, or **plant insulin**. It is believed that bitter melon acts on both the pancreas and in nonpancreatic cells, such as muscle cells.Bitter Melon has been shown to reduce cholesterol and triglycerides.In Brasil it is used for cancer,wounds rheumatism,malaria,and diabetes .

Black Seed: Black seed Oil (Nigella Sativa) - Also called black cumin seed. Blackseed oil is legendary for its medicinal properties and has been used for thousands of years Preliminary research in animal trials has shown that that an extract from Nigella sativa seeds can reduce elevated blood sugar levels and the antioxidant activity of the extract may prevent the complications associated with uncontrolled type

Chapter IXV

II diabetes. It was narrated by Prophet Muhammad (Peace be upon Him) that **Black seed is a cure for all diseases except death.**

Blueberry: Blueberry leaves have traditionally been used to control blood sugar levels when they are slightly elevated - Sugar results have shown that the leaves have an active ingredient with a remarkable ability to get rid the body of excessive sugar in the blood. It is a good astringent and helps relieve inflammation of the kidney, bladder and prostate.

Chili Peppers: *From The 50 Miracle Cures of Coriander Book by Professor Awad Mansour:*

Chili peppers lower blood sugar and protect the heart. The main active compound in all chili peppers, from cayenne to jalapeño, is capsaicin, the spice that gives curry powder its heat. According to an Australian study published in the American Journal of Clinical Nutrition, eating hot curry, such as vindaloo, helps lower glucose levels while supporting the liver and pancreas (one reason, perhaps, that hot curries are so popular as a late-night meal in Britain .

The antioxidants in capsaicin help combat free radicals, thereby cutting down on chronic inflammation in the body, a precursor to diabetes, arthritis and other chronic illnesses. A study of 27 adults found that eating fresh chilis minimized oxidation of cells that, under certain conditions, leads to damaging free radicals, chronic inflammation and disease.

Arthritis sufferers already know that capsaicin cream relieves sore joints, but it is also effective in treating sensory nerve disorders, such as diabetic neuropathy. And by helping to reduce blood cholesterol and triglycerides, capsaicin also helps prevent platelet clumping that can predispose diabetics to heart attacks and stroke.

Chilis are high in vitamin C and carotenoids, which help regulate insulin. Two teaspoons of chili peppers provide 6% of your recommended DV(daily vitamin) for vitamin C and 10% of the DV for vitamin A — vitamins that help repair the compromised immune systems of diabetics. Chilis also help you lose weight. That's because their searing heat in the mouth burns energy, and therefore calories.

Cinnamon: One of the world's most famous spice and herbal remedy through centuries. It is native to India.It was used for colds,flu,vomiting, diarrhea. The combination of honey and cinnamon has been used in both oriental and Ayurvedic medicine for centuries for heart disease,arthritis,hair loss,toothache,bladder infection,cholesterol, indigestion,colds,acne,obesity,hypertension,diabetes,infertility,immunes ystem and,cancer It was reported to augment the insulin action , lower both blood sugar and high blood pressure as well as high cholesterol. The active ingredient in cinnamon was at first thought to be MHCP but in 2004 Dr Anderson stated that that was incorrect and the real ingredient causing the changes was the water soluble polyphenol type-A polymer.

CINNAMON IS THE BEST SPICE FOR DIABETES

This benefit was confirmed in a study conducted at University of California, Santa Barbara. A half of a teaspoon of cinnamon significantly dropped the blood sugar levels in 60 diabetic participants.

Over the years, people have discovered the source of cinnamon and, with the advent of technology, acquiring cinnamon is no longer very difficult.Medical experts have been studying the health benefits that one can get from the consumption of cinnamon. One case to prove that point is a recent randomized, placebo-controlled, double-blind study conducted by researchers from London's Imperial College regarding the benefits of cinnamon on diabetes patients.

Cinnamon and Diabetes: Is there a link?

In order to find the association between cinnamon and its effects on patients with diabetes, a group of researchers from the Imperial College in London, headed by Dr. Akilen, conducted a study which involved 58 patients diagnosed with type 2 diabetes and whose mean age was 55. Each participant was randomly assigned to either of two groups: one group received a supplement of 2 grams of cinnamon every day, and another group received placebo. The length of time wherein the participants received the intervention was 12 weeks. After the study, the results revealed that the intake of cinnamon supplement was linked to an average **decrease in systolic blood pressure** of 3.4 mmHg, and a decrease in **diastolic blood pressure** of 5.0 mmHg. As for the results of the placebo group, no significant reduction in blood pressure was noted.

When it comes to the participants' blood sugar level, the researchers noticed a decrease in glycated haemoglobin levels ,A1c,over twelve weeks in the cinnamon group – from 8.22 percent to 7.86 percent. In the placebo group, on the other hand, researchers noted an increase in A1c levels – from 8.55 percent to 8.68 percent over a period of twelve weeks. A1c is used in measuring the levels of sugar in the blood.

Health Benefits of Cinnamon

It helps lower bad cholesterol (LDL) levels. Studies have shown that it has the ability to stop yeast infections that have become resistant to medications.A study conducted by researchers from the U.S. Department of Agriculture located in Maryland revealed that cinnamon reduced the propagation of lymphoma and leukaemia cancer cells. Cinnamon is said to prevent the formation of blood clots.A study conducted at the Copenhagen University revealed that patients who were given half teaspoon of cinnamon powder mixed with one tablespoon of honey each morning prior to eating breakfast experienced a significant relief in pain brought about by arthritis after one week. Another study indicated that inhaling the smell of cinnamon helps boost memory and cognitive function. Ordinary cinnamon has drug-like powers to remove excess glucose from your bloodstream.

The latest results came from Kansas State University, where researchers carried out tests on unpasteurised apple juice. In the US, such juice has been linked to at least one outbreak of the disease in which a girl died and 66 people fell ill.They found that one teaspoon of cinnamon added to the juice **killed 99.5 per cent of the bacteria** within three days. Last year, the same researchers added spices to raw ground beef and sausage. They found that **cinnamon, clove and garlic were the most powerful in killing E.coli.**

Coccinia indica (Ivy gourd): East Indian traditional medicine uses this plant to treat "urine sugar". People take it in powder or in dried pellet form. Ivy gourd appears to imitate the action of insulin in the body.

In clinical studies, Ivy gourd lowered blood glucose in people with type 2 diabetes, with no adverse effects.

Cordyceps Sinensis Mushroom: Researchers from University of Macau, China, isolated a polysaccharide of molecular weight approximately 210kDa was isolated from cultured Cordyceps mycelia. This isolated polysaccharides, CSP-1, has a strong antidant activity and a hypoglycemic effect on normal and alloxan-diabetic mice and streptozotocin (STZ)-diabetic rats. When administered at a dose of higher than 200mg/kg body wt. daily for 7 days, CSP-1 produced a significant drop in blood glucose level in both STZ-induced diabetic rats and alloxan-induced diabetic mice. Researchers from China Agricultural University, Beijing, also noticed the blood glucose lowering effects of a polysaccharide extracted from the fruting bodies and mycelia of Cordyceps militaris in a study of rats. The hypoglycemic effect of this polysaccharide- enriched Cordyceps militaris extract was dose-dependent.

Cordyceps Sinensis is famous for other health benefits ; for cancer,immunity,liver,heart,memory, asthma,high blood pressure,male sex,energy,cholesterol and as anti-ager.

Coriander: *From: The 50 Miracle Cures of Coriander Book by Professor Awad Mansour:*

Coriander helps reduce blood sugar levels. Coriander is a potent curry spice that's beneficial for people with diabetes. The fresh plant is pungent. It's known by its Mexican name of cilantro in America and generally chopped and used in salsas, salads and other dishes. In India and other countries, both the plant and its dried seeds are known as coriander. As a pantry item, it's easiest to buy it as whole seeds or ground and use as needed.

Coriander helps reduce blood sugar levels by promoting the release of insulin from the pancreas, so that glucose can be used by the cells. Both the fresh leaves of the cilantro plant (which is very popular in Mexican cooking) and its dried seeds are high in phytonutrients, flavonoids and polyphenols. These include quercetin, which protects against cardiovascular disease and eye problems such as retinopathy, associated with diabetes.

Chapter IXV

Elecampane: Elecampane is obtained from the dried cut root and rhizomes of lnula helenium. Elecampane compounds may exhibit variable antiseptic, antibacterial, antifungal, diuretic, expectorant, and hypotensive activities. Elecampane is used to treat **diabetes,** hypertension, diseases of the respiratory tract such as bronchitis, asthma, and cough, diseases of the GI tract, and diseases of the kidney and lower urinary tract. It's also used to stimulate appetite and bile production, to treat dyspepsia and menstrual complaints, and to promote dieresis .Also it is excellent for most skin disorders.

Figs Leaf : Victor Marchione, MD wrote: Fig leaves are healing foods that are best known as an effective alternative therapy for treating diabetes.In one clinical trial, researchers from the Faculty of Medicine, University Hospital, Madrid, Spain, studied the effects of a decoction of fig leaves ("Ficus carica") on diabetes control. Six men and four women who were insulin-dependent diabetes patients were recruited for the trial. The patients were managed with their usual diabetes diet and their twice-daily insulin injection. During the first month, patients were given a decoction of fig leaves; during the next month, they were given a non-sweet commercial tea.

In addition to their anti-diabetic properties, figs leaves have strong antioxidant and anti-inflammatory properties. In a clinical trial conducted at the Faculty of Pharmacy, New Delhi, India, researchers evaluated the anti-inflammatory and antioxidant activity of "F. carica" leaves. Their study validated that the antioxidant effect of fig leaves is likely due to the presence of steroids and flavonoids and the anti-inflammatory activity could be due to free radical scavenging activity.

KELP :A study was conducted at the University of Hanyang in South Korea 2008 showed that eating kelp powder decreased blood sugar. It is very beneficial for people who suffer with low thyroid function, pregnant women and people on a low salt diet. This seaweed contains 23 minerals, including chlorophyll, folic acid, vitamins A, B12, D and iodine.Sea Kelp provides many health benefits such as: *brittle nails and hair,obesity,constipation,dry skin,fatigue, increased blood cholesterol levels,cold hands and feet,poor concentration and memory,enlarged* *thyroid gland,kills herpes virus,hair loss,poor digestion,bowl gas and anemia.*

IODINE FOR DIABETES: It was while treating a large 320-pound woman with insulin dependent diabetes that we learned a valuable lesson regarding the role of Iodine in hormone receptor function. This woman had come in via the emergency room with a very high random blood sugar of 1,380 mg/dl. She was then started on insulin during her hospitalization and was instructed on the use of a home glucometer. She was to use her glucometer two times per day. Two weeks later on her return office visit for a checkup of her insulin dependent diabetes she was informed that during her hospital physical examination she was noted to have FBD. She was recommended to start on 50 mg of iodine(4 tablets) at that time. One week later she called us requesting to lower the level of insulin due to having problems with hypoglycemia. She was told to continue to drop her insulin levels as long as she was experiencing hypoglycemia and to monitor her blood sugars carefully with her glucometer. Four weeks later during an office visit her glucometer was downloaded to my office computer, which showed her to have an average random blood sugar of 98. I praised the patient for her diligent efforts to control her diet and her good work at keeping her sugars under control with the insulin. She then informed me that she had come off her insulin three weeks earlier and had not been taking any medications to lower her blood sugar. When asked what she felt the big change was, she felt that her diabetes was under better control due to the use of iodine."

Iodine is a key element in fighting diabetes because it helps regulate the thyroid and is essential for a healthy liver, gallbladder, pancreas, spleens and more. While it is well known that diet, obesity, food allergies, viral infections, and stress are all contributing factors for diabetes, it is less widely recognized that these factors are often either a cause of or caused by a weak liver, spleen, and pancreas.

In women, iodine's ability to revive hormonal sensitivity back to normal significantly improves Insulin sensitivity and other hormones.

Chapter IXV

For diabetes, take at least 50 mg per day of Iodine (a combination of both elemental and potassium iodide) and selenium must also be taken in order for iodine to work properly.

Gingko Biloba: Long used in traditional Chinese medicine, The extract may prove useful for prevention and treatment of early-stage diabetic neuropathy. Gingko Biloba extract improves blood flow in the peripheral tissues of the nerves in the arms, legs, hands, and feet and is therefore an important medicine in the treatment of peripheral vascular disease. It has also been shown to prevent diabetic retinopathy.

Green Banana Peels - Wash a green plantain and peel it, then put the peel in a jar and cover with water. Let sit overnight, and then drink this water three times a day to lower your blood sugar level. Keep drinking as needed and change the peel every other day and refill the jar with water.

Goat's Rue(The Natural Metformin): Goat's rue, sometimes called Holy Hay,it is indigenous to southern Europe and western Asia and was first mentioned by dairy farmer Gillet-Damitte in 1873 in a letter to the French Academy in which he described milk production increases in his cows of between 35-50 percent when given this herb. In addition to its lactogenic properties, goat's rue comes from the same family as fenugreek and is also considered to have anti-diabetic properties. Goat's Rue contains galegine, a guanidine compound from which phenformin, the precursor drug to metformin (Glucophage), was derived. Metformin is considered an insulin receptor sensitizer and one anti-aging researcher believes that it may have a beneficial effect on other resistant hormone receptors as well. Because metformin has been found beneficial in many cases of polycystic ovary syndrome, goat's rue may be an especially appropriate galactogogue herb as it may have properties that address underlying problems.

A 1999 study also reported a weight-loss effect of goat's rue upon mice (test amount used was 10% of dietary weight) that was associated with the lowering of glucose. Other benefits of Goat's Rue are:It increases production and flow of milk ,Reduces blood sugar levels,Promotes sweating, and Increases urine output .

Green Tea: Green tea,also known as Chinese tea ,has been a popular beverage in Asia for 3000 years.About 60 years ago,Dr.Minowada of Kyoto University noticed urine sugar was reduced when patients used green tea.Green tea contains catechins and polysaccharides which are responsible for lowring blood sugar.Green tea has many other benefits for cancer,cholesterol,high blood pressure and skin disorders.

Gymnema Sylvestre(Sugar Destroyer): Native to India, also known as **Gurmar** which means the "**sugar destroyer**". To treat diabetes, dried leaves are pounded together with coriander fruit ,juice is extracted and given orally. This remedy has been used in India for treating diabetes for about 2000 years. Today in India it is being used to treat primarily type II diabetes and type I as well. Gymnema also improves the ability of insulin to lower blood sugar in both type I and type II diabetes.

EVIDENCE OF A MIRACLE

In 1990 a series of published studies on Gymnema Sylvestre Extract lifted this herb from interesting to revolutionary. To begin with, it was shown that the administration of Gymnema Sylvestre Extract to diabetic animals not only resulted in improved glucose homeostasis, this improvement was accompanied by regeneration of beta cells in the pancreas.

In the words of researchers, " This herbal therapy appears to bring about blood glucose homeostasis through increased serum insulin levels provided by repair/regeneration of the endocrine pancreas.

" To my knowledge, this is the only compound that has shown the ability to lessen indicators of diabetes by directly repairing/regenerating the pancreas cells responsible for producing insulin".

As abnormalities in beta cell number and/or function are directly related to both Type I (insulin dependent) and Type II diabetes mellitus, it appeared that Gymnema Sylvestre(GS) Extract was a major discovery in the battle against one of the most common disorders in the world.

Chapter IXV

Also in 1990, this same research team published results on their treatment of both Type I and Type II diaetics and Gymnema Sylvestre Extract over a period of more than 2 years.

In the case if Type II diabetics, Gymnema Sylvestre Extract resulted in significant reductions in blood glucose, glycosylated hemoglobin, glycosylated plasma proteins, and conventional drug dosage.
At the beginning of the study all participants were taking oral antidiabetic medication, and treatment with Gymnema Sylvestre Extract resulted not only in a lowering of oral medication necessity, but almost 25% of the participants were able to discontinue conventional oral medication and maintain blood glucose homeostasis with GS Extract alone.

Additionally,GS Extract significantly improved cholesterol, triglyceride, and free fatty acid level's that were elevated in the study participants.

According to Dr. Baskaran and Dr. Ahamath, of the Department of Biochemistry, Post-Graduate Institute of Basic Medical Sciences, Madras, India, the therapeutic properties of Gymnema Sylvestre, an extract from the leaves of Gymnema Sylvestre, in controlling hyperglycaemia was investigated in 22 Type II diabetic patients on conventional oral anti-hyperglycaemic agents.

Fenugreek Seed: Fenugreek is a common well known herbal remedy in Africa, Asia and Middle East (by Egyptians,Greeks and Romans)for centuries.It was used for asthma, fevers, wounds, cholesterol, diabetes, ulcer and cancer. Fenugreek seeds were used as an oral insulin substitute and it is considered as a main pillar in treating diabetes. It lowers blood sugar by 34.8 percent and works miracles for cholesterol, too.

Garlic: Garlic is an ideal old herbal remedy.It is used by most nations for different types of infections,to reduce cholesterol, high blood pressure and blood sugar levels.Also it improves blood circulation and as an antioxidant due to its vitamin C and E content.

Allicin, alliin, garlic extract were tested on solid and ascites mouse tumors resulted in complete inhibition of tumor growth.

GARLIC OIL FOR DIABETES AND HEART

Scientists have found that garlic has "significant" potential for preventing a condition called "cardiomyopathy." This type of heart disease a leading cause of death in people with diabetes, making it a very significant health issue. The new study, which also explains why diabetics are at high risk for cardiomyopathy, appears in the Journal of Agricultural and Food Chemistry. The group of researchers had hints from past studies that garlic might protect against heart disease. And that garlic might help control the abnormally high blood sugar levels that occur in diabetes. But they realized that few studies had been done specifically on garlic's effects on "diabetic cardiomyopathy". They concluded that garlic oil possesses significant potential for protecting hearts at risk for this life-threatening disease.

Ginger: Ginger is an anti-inflammatory. Ginger is an antioxidant with powerful anti-inflammatory compounds called gingerols. A study published in Life Sciences found that gingerols inhibit the production of nitric oxide, which quickly forms a damaging free radical called peroxynitrite.

Ginger not only boosts the immune system but also helps soothe the digestive system. This is important for people with diabetes because elevated blood sugar tends to impair digestion and lead to gastrointestinal complications. In a study published in the Journal of Pharmacology and Experimental Therapeutics, ginger was found to reduce the negative effect of high blood sugar on the stomach's rhythm and rate of emptying. The researchers concluded that while bringing blood sugar down is Job One for people with diabetes, eating foods infused with large quantities of ginger, such as curry, helps improve digestion.

Glucomannan Konjac: Glucomannan is a water-soluble polysaccharide dietary fiber. It is also a food additive used as an emulsifier and thickener. This supplement is gaining popularity and consumers realize many health benefits it offers. Products containing

Chapter IXV

glucomannan, marketed under a variety of brand names, are sold as dietary supplements for constipation, obesity, high cholesterol, and type 2 diabetes. You will often find it in 500 mg and 600 mg capsules.

There have been many human studies evaluating the benefit of glucomannan on blood lipids, body weight, fasting blood glucose, and blood pressure. Most of the clinical trial show it lowered total cholesterol, LDL cholesterol, triglycerides, body weight, and fasting blood glucose. Glucomannan has a role to play in clinical medicine in terms of reducing total cholesterol, LDL cholesterol, triglycerides, fasting blood sugar, and perhaps body weight, but does not seem to have much of an effect on HDL cholesterol or blood pressure.

Konjac Glucomannan was proven to lower serum thyroid hormones in hyperthyroidis.(From:J Am Coll Nutr. 2007. Istanbul University, Istanbul Faculty of Medicine).

Holy Basil (Tulsi): Traditionally, this sacred herb native to the Indian subcontinent was used to treat colds and flue, gas, nausea, pain and arthritis.It has also been shown to have antioxidant and anti-inflammatory properties, and as such may be able to ward off cancer and protect the body from damage.

However recently many researchers are focusing on a holy basil cholesterol and diabetes treatment, as the herb has shown some promise in treating both of these conditions.

Studies have illustrated that the holy basil plant has cholesterol lowering properties, as well as the ability to reduce triglyceride levels. Holy basil has similar effects to diabetes medications, and may mimic the effects of insulin in the body.

Neem: For centuries the Neem tree has been known as the wonder tree of India. It's a tree that is very versatile as far as medical benefits are concerned. All parts of neem including seeds, leaves, flowers and bark have medicinal properties. It offers plenty of usages in several shapes and sizes. It has anti-fungal, anti-bacterial, anti-viral, and anti-diabetic properties.

137

Each and every part of neem tree is being used and it has lots of health benefits. Below are the some of the benefits that neem possesses:

1. **Cure Eczema:** Recent studies indicate that neem leaf extracts (in form of a Soap or shampoo containing Neem oil) can easily relieve the itching and redness of eczema. To obtain the benefits of neem, you can take a warm bath with neem leaves in it. The neem bath heals and protects you from any minor skin infections.

2. **Effective Detoxification:** It works as blood purifier and is very helpful in eradicating toxins from the blood. It also helps making our immune system very strong and efficient to fight against any foreign invasion.

3. **Dental care:** The twig of neem tree is largely used as a tooth brush in different regions of India, Pakistan and Bangladesh. This keeps the teeth whiter and prevents gum problems. Neem is also used to treat bad breath, tooth decay, bleeding and sore gums and to prevent cavities. Hence, it is an important ingredient in a variety of oral care products sold worldwide.

4. **Good for Digestion:** Neem tea is an effective tonic for both indigestion and constipation because of the content of tict rasa. Eating neem will help get rid of intestinal worms, thus performing its role as a de-worming agent. It also eliminates the problem of acidity. It is highly recommended in hyperacidity and epigastric pain.

5. **Effective against diabetes:** Diabetes is a disease of excess sweetness so bitter herbs and foods must be used to counteract the imbalance. Neem has been shown to control blood sugar levels and prevent adrenaline as well as glucose induced hyperglycaemia.

6. **Effective against Arthritis:** The pain, inflammation, and swelling of the joints in arthritis can be greatly reduced by massaging muscle aches and joints with Neem oil. In addition to its anti-inflammatory effects there are several compounds like polysaccharides, catechin, and limonoids present in neem that act as pain killers.

7. **Anti cancer:** The polysaccharides and limonoids found in Neem not only reduce the tumors and cancers but are also effective against lymphocytic leukemia. Another protein found in the neem leaf has been found to boost the immune response and helps to kill colon cancer cells.

8. **Skin care:** Neem leaves paste when mixed with fresh turmeric (haldi) and applied to the face, clears the face of pimples and also reduces scars. Dry skin, dandruff, itchy scalp, wrinkles, skin ulcers and other conditions that can be effectively resolved by the use of soaps, lotions, and creams, containing Neem leaf extracts and oil.

9. **Anti bacterial:** Neem oil contains powerful antiviral and antibacterial properties that make it the first choice in over a hundred household, agricultural, medicinal and cosmetic products. Infections caused by bacteria (such as acne) or fungus (such as jock itch) are both curable by using neem oil. To kill germs and bacteria on your skin, boil some neem leaves in water regularly and use the water to wash your body.

10. **Anti malaria:** Neem usage boosts the body's immune system making a person less likely to contract malaria and more likely to heal faster if he does. Since neem also acts as a natural pesticide, it repels mosquitoes which primarily carry malarial infection.

11. **Hair health:** When used as hair oil, neem promotes shiny, healthy hair, combats dryness, prevents premature graying and may even help with some forms of hair loss.

12. **Contraceptive properties:** Modern research suggests that neem does indeed kill sperm within seconds after contact and that the protection lasts for five hours. It is a safe and effective method of birth control, with no side effects. On top of preventing pregnancy, it may also protect from some sexually transmitted diseases.

Nopal (Prickly Pear Cactus): Dried powder from Prickly Pear Cactus is taken in capsule form. The plant has a high soluble fiber content that may reduce glucose absorption by the intestines. Two controlled short-term studies in people with type 2 diabetes reported lowered fasting blood glucose and increased insulin sensitivity. There were no side effects noted.

Oleander Leaf :Oleander Extract- A carefully prepared aqueous extract of the oleander plant made according to the directions in the book "Cancer's Natural Enemy" by Tony M. Isaacs (which also contains 20% Sutherlandia frutescens, the famed "South Africa Cancer Bush") online at http://www.sutherlandia.opc. Diabetics who have used this remedy report being able to either reduce or eliminate medications altogether, often being able to control their diabetes with diet alone. Note: Oleander is highly toxic in raw form, but safe when boiled and strained according to the directions in the book.

Olive Leaf: Olive leaf (Olea europaea) was first used medicinally in Ancient Egypt. It is gaining recognition as a powerful defender against sickness and numerous scientific studies have been conducted to investigate the extract's beneficial properties. The reported benefits of olive leaf extract range from promoting increased energy and healthy blood pressure, to supporting the cardiovascular system and the immune system.

Olives are native to Asia Minor and Syria, but are cultivated in Mediterranean countries and also Chile, Peru and South Australia. More recent knowledge of the olive leaf's medicinal properties dates back to the early 1800s when pulverised leaves were used in a drink to lower fevers. A few decades later, green olive leaves were used in tea as a treatment for malaria.

From research and clinical experience to date, we can say that supplemental olive leaf may be beneficial in the treatment for conditions caused by, or associated with, a virus ,bacterium or protozoan. Among those treatable conditions are: influenza, the common cold, candida infections, meningitis, Epstein-Barr virus (EBV), herpes I and II, human herpes virus 6 and 7, shingles (Herpes zoster), HIV/ARC/AIDS, chronic fatigue, hepatitis B, pneumonia, tuberculosis, gonorrhea, malaria, dengue, severe diarrhea, and dental, ear, urinary tract ,high blood pressure, obesity, diabetes and surgical infections.

140

Chapter IXV

Onion: Onion is a member of the lily family (Liliaceae). It is native to Eurasia but now grows all over the world, due mostly to people bringing it with them as a staple food wherever they migrated. Experimental and clinical evidence suggests that onion consists of an active ingredient called APDS (allyl propyl disulphide). APDS has been shown to block the breakdown of insulin by the liver and possibly to stimulate insulin production by the pancreas, thus increasing the amount of insulin and reducing sugar levels in the blood.

Pterocarpus Marsupium:(also known as Indian Kino, in English) is a large deciduous tree. Commonly grows in central, western, and southern parts of India and Sri Lanka. Pterocarpus marsupium demonstrates to reduce the glucose absorption from the gastrointestinal tract, and improve insulin and pro-insulin levels. It also effective in beta cell regeneration for type 1 diabetes . The heartwood of pterocarpus marsupium is astringent, bitter acrid, anti inflammatory. It is considered magical for diabetes. It turns the water blue as soon as it comes in contact with the water. It is good for elephantiasis, leucoderma, diarrhoea, dysentery, rectalgia, cough and greyness of hair. The bark is used as an astringent and in toothache.The bruised leaves are considered useful as an external application for boils, sores and skin diseases.

Pycnogenol: is a powerful antioxidant derived from French maritime **pine tree bark** and the subject of more than 180 studies over 35 years which has been shown to reduce high blood pressure, LDL cholesterol and blood glucose without affecting insulin levels. Of particular note is its ability to reduce leakage into the retina by repairing capillaries in the eyes. While still largely unknown to American doctors, Pycnogenol is the leading prescription for diabetic retinopathy in France. A New study discovers how Pycnogenol lowers blood glucose levels in type 2 diabetes ;Pycnogenol delays glucose absorption 190 times more potently than prescription medications.

In two separate studies conducted in 2004, Pycnogenol® was found to significantly lower blood sugar levels in type II diabetes patients. This study opens new avenues for Pycnogenol® in the field of diabetes, metabolic syndrome and obesity.

Salacia Oblonga: The traditional Indian herbal called Salacia Oblonga has been found by U.S. researchers to lower blood and insulin responses after eating.

As reported in the American Journal of Clinical Nutrition: The extract of Salacia oblonga lowers acute glycemia and insulinemia in persons with type 2 diabetes after a high-carbohydrate meal. The results from this study suggest that Salacia may be beneficial to this population for postprandial glucose control."The said study was conducted by Researchers from Abbott Laboratories and Radiant Research and found that Salacia oblonga acts in a similar way to diabetes medications: by binding to intestinal enzymes calledalpha-glucosidases.Alpha-glucosidases are the enzymes responsible for breaking down carbohydrates into glucose. In the presence of the herbal extract, the enzyme binds to the herbal extract rather than a carbohydrate, thereby resulting to less glucose getting into the blood stream - thus lowering blood glucose and insulin levels. Results of the abovementioned randomised, double-blinded crossover study showed that both doses (240 or 480 mg) of the herbal significantly lowered the postprandial glucose response by 14 and 22 per cent for the 240 mg and 480 mg extract, respectively, compared to the control meal. It also shows hepatoprotective effects and also used as liver tonic. It is effective in case of rheumatism, skin diseases and inflammation.

Shilajit – Destroyer of Diabetes?: If you are diabetic and are looking for a natural alternative to lower and effectively control your blood sugar levels, then you may be in luck. An herb-like substance derived from the high altitudes of the Himalayan Mountains, shilajit, has been used for centuries to prevent and combat numerous health problems, including diabetes.

For centuries, shilajit has been called the "destroyer of weakness." Now some researchers in India are calling it the "destroyer of diabetes." : Research was conducted at the Medical College in Baroda, India, with the specific purpose of studying the effects of shilajit on blood glucose and lipid profiles in diabetic rats as well its effects when combined with conventional anti-diabetic drugs. Using albino rats, the study design included measuring blood glucose levels, total cholesterol, triglyceride and high-density lipoproteins before and after treatment. Each group of rats were given different amounts of shilajit, either by itself or given with other anti-diabetic drugs such as metformin.

The results? Across the board, each group of rats given shilajit experienced a reduction in blood glucose levels as well as a significant increase in the HDL level. Positive changes in the rats lipid profile is understandable given the derangement of glucose, fat and protein metabolism which occurs when one has diabetes. Thus the researchers from the Medical College in Baroda(1) concluded that shilajit is a legitimate, natural supplement that can help in the long-term management of those effected with diabetes.

Benefits of Shilajit / Uses of Shilajit:

The following are some of the most important reasons for which Shilajit has gained its worldwide renown today:-

(i) Aphrodisiacal Properties : Shilajit is known best in India for its aphrodisiacal properties. Its mention has been made even in the great Indian treatise of sex, Kama Sutra, written by Vatsyayana. Shilajit can increase libido in both men and women. It is used worldwide in the treatment of impotence, erectile dysfunction, low sperm count, premature ejaculation, etc.

(ii) Chest Problems :Medical science has proved conclusively that Shilajit is useful in treating several problems of the chest. It is used in the treatment of allergies and in the treatment of respiratory disorders such as bronchitis, colds, cough, pneumonia, emphysema, etc.

(iii) Diabetes Mellitus: Due to its properties as a panacea, Shilajit is widely used in the treatment of diabetes. It carries the sugars in the blood to their final destination.

(iv) Nervous Disorders: Shilajit is potent in the treatment of nervous disorders.

(v) Obesity :Shilajit has the capacity to break down fat that has accumulated in the body.

(vi) Vigor and Vitality: Shilajit is very popularly prescribed for its very beneficial effects in enhancing vigor and vitality

Dr. Mansour

Traditionally Shilajit is considered a panacea for kidney disorders, it increases the core energy responsible for your sexual and spiritual power, the same force that is withered by stress and anxiety. It is used by the indigenous system of medicine in India, Hakims and traditional healers, in a great variety of diseases: genitourinary diseases, diabetes, chronic bronchitis, asthma, gall stones, jaundice, painful and bleeding piles, enlarged liver and spleen, fermentative dyspepsia, digestive disorders, worms, renal and bladder calculi, nervous debility, sexual neurasthenia, hysteria, anemia and in bone fracture. It is also used for Female infertility, Obesity , Joint pains, Wounds, and chronic ulcers, Skin diseases, Elephantiasis, Facial paralysis, Nasal ulcers......

Syzygium Cumini(Java Plum or Jambolan)Fruit: Evergreen Indian tree which was proven in a number of studies to regenerate beta cells in the pancreas and it does lower the cumulative sugar value A1C for type 1 and 2 diabetes. Reductions on blood sugar levels by about 30% seem reasonably to be expected. The bark has anti-inflammatory activity and is used In India for anemia, the bark and seed for diabetes which reduce the blood sugar level quickly, the fruit for dysentery and leave's juice for gingivitis (bleeding gums).Syzygium Cumini the fruit has properties anti-stringent, stomach, carminative, antiscorbutic and diuretic and the leaves and the fruits are used in diverse forms to do that the natural treatments for a very ample variety of problems like the diarrhea, the diabetes, the ringworms and many more.

Turmeric: The active ingredient in turmeric is **curcumin**. Tumeric has been used for over 2500 years in India, where it was most likely first used as a dye.

The medicinal properties of this spice have been slowly revealing themselves over the centuries. Long known for its anti-inflammatory properties, recent research has revealed that turmeric is a natural wonder, proving beneficial in the treatment of many different health conditions from cancer to Alzheimer's disease.

Professor Mansour discussed 50 health benefits of curcumin in his book:The 50 Miracle Cures of Curcumin: Here are some benefits of them: *It is a natural antiseptic and antibacterial agent, useful in disinfecting cuts,wounds, and burns,acne,psoriasis,arthritis,diabetes,liver*

144

cirrhosis, renal failure,all types of cancer, ulcer, asthma,urinary tract infection, cholesterol ,memory, multiple sclerosis, weight loss, depression.

Curcumin is available now in 500-1000 mg capsules

RAIN FOREST AMAZON TROPICAL HERBS

Agaricus Blazei Murrill (ABM) Mushroom : Referred to in it's native Brazil as "The Mushroom of the Gods" with good reason due to it's amazing immune boosting and disease fighting properties. **Agaricus blazei** is an edible mushroom native to Brazil and cultivated in Japan for its medicinal uses. In vitro experiments and studies done in mice have shown that Agaricus has immunomodulatory, antitumor, and antimutagenic properties. Agaricus Blazei Murill has been used to treat **arteriosclerosis, hepatitis, hyperlipidemia, diabetes, dermatitis**, and **cancer**. The polysaccharides and anti-angiogenic compounds present in Agaricus are thought to be responsible for its antitumor properties. Such effects are believed to be exerted by **immunopotentiation** or **direct inhibition of angiogenesis**..A recent randomized study showed that oral administration of Agaricus extract improved the natural killer cell activity and quality of life in gynecological **cancer patients undergoing chemotherapy**. However, more studies are needed to confirm these observations. Agaricus blazei was also shown to have **antidiabetic** effects in vitro and in animal studies. In addition, results from a study done in human subjects with Type 2 diabetes suggest benefits of agaricus extract in **improving insulin resistance**.

Cashew Leaf and Bark: The natural rainforest remedy for diarrhea and dysentery is 1/2 cup of a standard decoction of leaves and twigs, taken two or three times daily.In Brazil it is used for : for asthma, bronchitis, corns, cough, **diabetes**, dyspepsia, eczema, fever, genital disorders, impotence, intestinal colic, leishmaniasis, libido stimulation, muscular debility, pain, psoriasis, scrofula, syphilis, throat (sore), tonsillitis, ulcers (mouth), urinary disorders, urinary insufficiency, venereal disease, warts, wounds, and used as a gargle and mouthwash.In Africa it is used for malaria.

Cat's Claw: is native to the Amazon. Used by indigenous tribes in Peru and South America to treat diabetes. Cat's claw has a long history of traditional use by indigenous peoples in South America. It has been used to treat digestive problems, arthritis, inflammation, ulcers,cancers,high blood pressure,HIV, and to promote wound healing.

Mullaca : is employed in herbal medicine systems today in both Peru and Brazil. In Peruvian herbal medicine the plant is called mullaca. To treat diabetes, the roots of three mullaca plants are sliced and macerated in 1/4 liter of rum for seven days. Honey is added, and 1/2 glass of this medicine is taken twice daily for 60 days. In addition, an infusion of the leaves is recommended as a good diuretic, and an infusion of the roots is used to treat hepatitis. For asthma and malaria, the dosage is 1 cup of tea made from the aerial parts of the plant. In Brazilian herbal medicine the plant is employed for chronic rheumatism, for skin diseases and dermatitis, as a sedative and diuretic, for fever and vomiting, and for many types of kidney, liver, diabetes,and gallbladder problems.

Pata de vaca: is native to South America .Pata de vaca's ability to lower blood sugar was first reported by a Brazilian researcher in an *in vivo* 1929 clinical study. In the mid-1980s, pata de vaca's continued use as a natural insulin substitute was reiterated in two Brazilian studies. Both studies reported *in vivo* hypoglycemic actions in various animal and human models. Chilean research in 1999 reported the actions of pata de vaca in diabetic rats. Their study determined that pata de vaca was found to "elicit remarkable hypoglycemic effects," and brought about a "decrease of glycemia in alloxan diabetic rats by 39%." In 2002, two *in vivo* studies on the blood-sugar-lowering effects of pata de vaca were conducted by two separate research groups in Brazil. The first study reported "a significant blood glucose-lowering effect in normal and diabetic rats." In the second study, 150 g of the leaf (per liter of water) was given to diabetic rats as their drinking water. Researchers reported that, after one month, those receiving pata de vaca had a "significant reduction in serum and urinary glucose and urinary urea . . ." as compared to the control group.

In 2004, a research group reported that pata de vaca again lowered blood sugar in rats and also reduced triglycerides, total cholesterol and HDL-cholesterol levels in diabetic rats stating, "These results suggest the validity of the clinical use of N. forficate in the treatment of diabetes mellitus type II. Other Brazilian researchers reported in 2004 that pata de vata, as well as a single chemical extracted from the leaves called *kaempferitrin*, significantly lowered blood sugar in diabetic rats at all dosages but lowered blood sugar in normal rats only at the highest dosages. They also documented an antioxidant effect. Toxicity studies published in 2004 indicate there were no toxic effects in either normal or diabetic rats, including pregnant diabetic rats.

Brazilian scientists have documented leaf extracts of pedra hume caá with hypoglycemic activity since 1929. Two clinical studies published in the 1990s again demonstrated its hypoglycemic activity and confirmed its traditional use for diabetes. In a 1990 double-blind placebo clinical study with normal and Type II diabetic patients, pedra hume caá (3 g powdered leaf daily) demonstrated the ability to lower plasma insulin levels in the diabetic group. In a 1993 study, 250 mg/kg of a leaf extract demonstrated the ability to reduce appetite and thirst, and to reduce urine volume, urinary excretion of glucose and urea in diabetic rats. The extract also inhibited the intestinal absorption of glucose. This study concluded that "aqueous extracts of Myrcia have a beneficial effect on the diabetic state, mainly by improving metabolic parameters of glucose homeostasis."

Stevia: For hundreds of years, indigenous peoples in Brazil and Paraguay have used the leaves of stevia as a sweetener. The Guarani Indians of Paraguay call it *kaa jheé* and have used it to sweeten their yerba mate tea for centuries. They have also used stevia to sweeten other teas and foods and have used it medicinally as a cardiotonic, for obesity, hypertension, and heartburn, and to help lower uric acid levels.

In addition to being a sweetener, stevia is considered (in Brazilian herbal medicine) to be hypoglycemic, hypotensive, diuretic, cardiotonic, and tonic. The leaf is used for diabetes, obesity, cavities, hypertension, fatigue, depression, sweet cravings, and infections. The leaf is employed in traditional medical systems in Paraguay for the same purposes as in Brazil.

Europeans first learned about stevia in the sixteenth century, when conquistadores sent word to Spain that the natives of South America were using the plant to sweeten herbal tea. Since then stevia has been used widely throughout Europe and Asia. In the United States, herbalists use the leaf for diabetes, high blood pressure, infections, and as a sweetening agent. In Japan and Brazil, stevia is approved as a food additive and sugar substitute. Brazilian scientists recorded stevioside's ability to lower systemic blood pressure in rats in 1991. Then in 2000, a double-blind, placebo-controlled study was undertaken with 106 Chinese hypertensive men and women.Therfore stevia is used as a safe zero-calorie sweetener,hypotensive and hypoglycemic for diabetes and high blood pressure.

Tetohuxtle Herbal Tea: is a tree bark tea that has been used, for hundreds of years, by the Indians in Mexico. It is derived from natural plants and is the best 100%natural alternative against DIABETES. The tea has also shown to be effective in helping with other symptoms like:Kidney problems, Cholesterol, Allergies, Fatigue, Numbness in toes and fingers, Loss of sexual functions and more.*It cleans the arteries helping to have one better circulation, to standardize the cholesterol, uric acid, and to clean the triglycerides; aid to prevent the blindness or loss of the view; it recovers the metabolism; it avoids that they appear the sores later and the external ulcers and recovers the damages caused by the Diabetes.*

VITAMINS FOR DIABETES

Vitamin B6 AND OTHER B VITAMINS FOR DIABETES

B vitamins are essential to health. Your nerves, skin, eyes, hair, liver, mouth, muscles, gastrointestinal tract, and brain depend on them for proper functioning. They are coenzymes that are involved in energy production and are also useful for alleviation of depression and anxiety.

As we get older our ability to absorb B vitamins from our food declines. In some Alzheimer's patients, it was found that the problem was due to a deficiency of vitamin B-12 plus vitamin B-complex in an accepted multivitamin.

The use of coffee, cigarettes, sugar and alcohol destroy B vitamins. People with diabetes and alcoholism need more B vitamins than most people. B vitamins are water-soluble and any excess is excreted and not stored in the body. Your body needs to replace B vitamins daily.

To get the most from your B's they should be taken as a group and the label should say "from whole foods" or "a whole food source". If you need more of a specific B vitamin such as B-12, add them along with the B-complex in your MULTIVITAMIN.

Many vitamin companies use bulk inorganic synthetic B-Complex vitamins, which our bodies cannot completely absorb. Food source or whole food Multivitamins are what you want to look for. If the label does not say food source on it, or from whole foods, then I would be concerned about the negative health value and the waste of money.

Symptoms of a Deficiency of B Vitamins:

Nausea, exhaustion, irritability, depression, forgetfulness, loss of appetite, weight gain, pain in muscles, poor immune response, loss of control of limbs, abnormal heart action, skin problems, acid reflux, splitting nails, mood swings, teary or bloodshot eyes etc.

Physical Problems:

Irregular Heart Beat, Acid Reflux, Migraine Headaches, Fatigue, Sore Mouth, Drowsiness, Dizziness, Headaches, Indigestion, Limbs Numb or Stiff, Limb pains, Abnormal Gait, Skin Eruptions, Labored Breathing, Low Blood Sugar, Soreness and Weakness in the Legs and Arms, Muscular Weakness, Reduced Sensory Perception, Difficulty Walking, Impotency in Men, Pernicious Anemia

Psychological Problems:

Mood Swings, Memory Loss, Difficulty Concentrating, Anxiety, Depression, Dementia, Emotional Sensitivity (can lead to asthma attacks), Loss of Mental Energy

Positive Benefits You May Notice While Taking Good B-Vitamins:

Increases body's ability to obtain oxygen, Helps extend cell lifespan, Regulates fat metabolism, Neutralizes the craving for liquor, Stimulates the bodies glandular and nervous systems, Lowers blood cholesterol and protein synthesis, Helpful in the treatment of heart disease and asthma, Very helpful to a smoker who is trying to quit, Important to residents in high-density pollution areas, Mellows the personality, Raises your ability to withstand stress, Relieves depression, Improves circulation and lowers cholesterol deposits in the skin and arteries to legs that restrict blood flow, Helpful in preventing heart attacks and strokes, Can help regulate blood sugar levels in hypoglycemic patients, Improves complexion (B3 or Niacin), Improves the production of hydrochloric acid for digestion, Improves the synthesis of sex hormones, Can relieve Hiatus Hernia, Can stop the craving for nicotine.

Be sure to get your B vitamins through a healthy diet or supplement with a natural B vitamin product.

Benfotiamine(Derived from Vitamin B1): A Supplement can reverse diabetic damage: Benfotiamine, a synthetic derivative of thiamine (vitamin B-1) which shows promise in treating a number of neurological and vascular conditions. Benfotiamine also appears to have beneficial anti-aging qualities, protecting human cells from harmful metabolic end products. Benfotiamine is not just for diabetics. With benfotiamine, the sustained increase of Thiamine Pyrophosphate (TPP) and the resulting activation of the enzyme transketolase in the system can produce beneficial effects on general nerve health, sciatica, neuropathy, retinopathy, nephropathy, polyneuropathy, peripheral neuropathy (PN), shingles, herpes zoster, fibromyalgia, general ageing, other nerve conditions, vascular health, blood pressure and coronary health for diabetics and non-diabetics alike.

Benfotiamine can effectively and safely elevate thiamine levels in the tissues and cells.

Benfotiamine (a lipid-soluble form of vitamin B-1) was developed in Japan in the late 1950's to treat alcoholic neuropathy, sciatica and other painful nerve conditions. It was patented in the U.S. in 1962, and has been in widespread use in Japan since 1962 and in Europe since 1978 with encouraging results and an excellent safety record.

Benfotiamine takes excess blood sugar and puts it to work -- restoring balance by allowing your blood cells to use the glucose instead of becoming overrun with the stuff. But that's not even close to all it does. It can actually reverse the damage caused by high blood sugar, including kidney and nerve damage. It's like getting your life back.

Chapter IXV ————————————————

Now, if Big Pharma would just start selling this stuff here in the United States, it would be a victory for diabetics!!because this is a rare case of a drug that works (even if it is just a synthetic vitamin).

Vitamin B9(Folic Acid): Scientists from China gave folic acid to mice with diabetes. Diabetes weakens blood vessels and can cause blood clots. In fact, most people who have diabetes don't die of too much sugar. They die of heart disease because the sugar's damaged their blood vessels.)

The scientists divided the diabetic mice into two groups. One group received a daily dose of folic acid. The second group of mice received no supplementation. After one month, scientists found that mice given folic acid reversed harmful damage (caused by diabetes) to the lining of their blood vessels. Scientists also saw marked improvements in a protein pathway that dilates blood vessels and prevents clotting. On the other hand, the mice not given folic acid did not experience these improvements

Vitamin C Competes with Glucose For Insulin Pumps:

Diabetics are probably not absorbing other nutrients from the blood as well. Vitamin C is structurally similar to glucose and the vitamin has a short half-life in the blood stream. It should concern medical professionals that vitamin C and glucose molecules share the same insulin-mediated tunneling mechanism into cells through the membrane.

In the 1970s, Emeritus Professor John T. A. Ely, University of Washington, proposed his Glucose-Ascorbate Antagonism (GAA) theory that predicts high glucose levels hinder vitamin C entry into cells. Animals which make their own vitamin C use dietary glucose as the raw material and the ascorbate and glucose molecules are similar. The similarity extends past molecular structure to the way they are attracted to, and enter, cells. Both molecules require help from the pancreatic hormone insulin before they can penetrate cell membranes using special "pumps." The name for the process that propels glucose and Vitamin C (the reduced form) through cell membranes is Insulin-mediated uptake.

Ely studied the insulin-mediated uptake of glucose and vitamin C using white blood cells. White blood cells have more insulin pumps and they may contain 20 times the amount of vitamin C as ordinary cells. Dr. Ely explains that both glucose and vitamin C molecules compete, but all things are not equal. The evolutionary "fight-or-flight" response favors glucose entry into cells at the expense of vitamin C. Because of this antagonism between sugar and Vitamin C, Ely recommends a low-carbohydrate, low-processed sugar diet.

Professor Ely told this author that he had advised Linus Pauling of the GAA theory and its prediction that Vitamin C would be less effective fighting colds in those who did not restrict their sugar intake. Recently, Ely and associates conducted a study on the common cold to test the GAA theory. Sugar and refined carbohydrates were restricted in the subjects. According to Dr. Ely, the remarkable (soon to be published) results showed an overwhelming preventive and curative property of vitamin C against the common cold in subjects with reduced sugar intake. (*Presumably these subjects did not suffer the cellular membrane malfunction commonly diagnosed as Diabetes Type II*).

The Diabetic Double Whammy

Combining these ideas, we postulate that cells that can't absorb glucose are not absorbing vitamin C either. As blood glucose levels rise, the GAA theory predicts that vitamin C uptake is greatly diminished throughout the body, even in cells with undamaged insulin pumps. Our conjecture is that the serious health consequences of prolonged Type II diabetes, e.g. blindness, wounds that won't heal, limb amputation, etc., are the result of the lack of vitamin C inside cells.

We may now more intelligently answer the question as to why heart patients do well on high-dose Omega-3 oil supplementation. Healthful omega-3 fatty acids, such as those found in flax seed and fish oils, promote healthy cell membranes allowing more nutrients to pass into cells. Theoretically, there would be more benefit from Omega-3 supplementation after the primary cause of membrane damage, trans fatty acids, are eliminated from the diet. As cell membranes become permeable, sugar molecules leave the blood stream lowering blood sugar, making vitamin C more bioavailable. Finally, we postulate that the cellular membrane problem hindering the uptake of glucose in diabetics also hinders their cells from obtaining vitamin C.

Chapter IXV

Heart patients, whose condition improves on Omega-3 oils, will improve even more as they eliminate processed foods, and follow Linus Paulings recommendation to increase their vitamin C dosage to individual bowel tolerance.

Stopping Diabetes Damage With Vitamin C

ScienceDaily (June 10, 2009) — Researchers at the Harold Hamm Oklahoma Diabetes Center have found a way to stop the damage caused by Type 1 diabetes with the combination of insulin and a common vitamin found in most medicine cabinets. While neither therapy produced desired results when used alone, the combination of insulin to control blood sugar together with the use of Vitamin C, stopped blood vessel damage caused by diabetes. The damage, known as endothelial dysfunction, is associated with most forms of cardiovascular disease such as hypertension, coronary artery disease, chronic heart failure, peripheral artery disease, diabetes and chronic renal failure.

By reducing or stopping the damage, patients with diabetes could avoid some of the painful and fatal consequences of the disease that include heart disease, reduced circulation and amputation, kidney disease and diabetic retinopathy, which can lead to blindness.

VITAMIN D3 AND DIABETES: Vitamin D influences more than 200 genes. This includes genes related to cancer and autoimmune diseases like multiple sclerosis.

Vitamin D affects your DNA through the vitamin D receptors (VDRs), which bind to specific locations of the human genome.

Reuters reports:"Vitamin D deficiency is a well-known risk factor for rickets, and some evidence suggests it may increase susceptibility to autoimmune diseases such as multiple sclerosis (MS), rheumatoid arthritis and type 1 diabetes, as well as certain cancers and even dementia."As a result, in the United States the late winter average vitamin D is only about 15-18 ng/ml, which is considered a very serious deficiency state.

In fact, new studies show that about 85 percent of the U.S. population is vitamin D deficient. This is primarily related to the recent appreciation that your levels of vitamin D should be MUCH higher than previously thought.

Consider the following vitamin D facts:

Vitamin D deficiency is epidemic in adults of all ages who have increased skin pigmentation, such as those whose ancestors are from Africa, the Middle East, or India, who always wear sun protection, or who limit their outdoor activities. African Americans and other dark-skinned people and those living in northern latitudes make significantly less vitamin D than other groups.

60 percent of patients with type 2 diabetes have vitamin D deficiency.

Studies showed very low levels of vitamin D among children, the elderly, and women;One nationwide study of women revealed that almost half of the African American women of childbearing age might be vitamin-D deficient.

Winter, when sun exposure is at its lowest, is the time of year when you need to be most concerned about the amount of vitamin D you are receiving, as your vitamin D levels can drop by up to 50 percent in the winter. Of course, if you have the tendency to spend the summer months indoors, out of the sun, or you only go outside with sunscreen on, then you would need to be concerned during the summer months as well.

The Many Health Benefits of Vitamin D

It's absolutely tragic that dermatologists and sunscreen manufacturers have done such a thorough job of deterring people from the sun -- your optimal source for natural vitamin D. **We noticed the fast results of psoriasis cases who took our psoriasis cream together with UV in our clinics in the Dead Sea area in Jordan since the UV Sun is the most balanced UV in the world.**

Their widely dispersed message to avoid the sun as much as possible, combined with an overall cultural trend of spending more time indoors during both work and leisure time, has greatly contributed to the widespread vitamin D deficiency seen today -- which in turn is fueling an astonishingly diverse array of common chronic diseases, including:

CANCER,Hypertension Heart disease ,Autism ,Obesity ,Rheumatoid arthritis ,Diabetes 1 and 2 Multiple Sclerosis, Crohn's disease ,Cold & Flu Inflammatory Bowel Disease Tuberculosis

Chapter IXV

,Septicemia Signs of aging Dementia ,Eczema & Psoriasis Insomnia Hearing loss ,Muscle pain Cavities Periodontal disease Osteoporosis Macular degeneration Reduced C-section risk ,Seizures, Infertility ,Asthma Cystic fibrosis Migraines ,Depression, Alzheimer's disease and Schizophrenia.

VITAMIN D3 IS A MUST FOR ALL DIABETICS

In this trial, 90 adults with type 2 diabetes were divided into three groups. Each group drank a yogurt beverage daily for 12 weeks. One group received plain yogurt, one received yogurt fortified with 500 IU of vitamin D, and the other group's yogurt contained 500 IU of D and extra calcium. Even the researchers were surprised by the results: Blood sugar levels in the plain yogurt group increased while sugar levels in both supplement groups dropped significantly.

More importantly, hemoglobin A1C went up in the plain group and down in the supplement groups. As I've shown you before, A1C gives an accurate assessment of blood sugar control over a span of several weeks.

Vitamin E*:* Vitamin E is associated with oils and oil-rich seeds and nuts. It is rare to find a fruit with significant amounts, except for the avocado and, now, kiwifruit. Kiwifruit actually has twice the vitamin E of avocado, but has only 60% of the avocado's calories.

A daily dose of Vitamin E may help delay the onset of type 2 diabetes in overweight adults at high risk of the disease, according to preliminary research.

Researchers in New Zealand found that high-dose Vitamin E appeared to temporarily improve insulin resistance - a precursor to type 2 diabetes - among adults, who were overweight.

"The results suggest that Vitamin E could have a role to play in delaying the onset of diabetes in at-risk individuals," said Dr. Patrick Manning and colleagues from the University of Otago in Dunedin in the journal diabetes Care .

This research supported the conclusions of recent studies, which found that people whose diets had a healthy dose of antioxidants, including Vitamin E, had a lower diabetes risk than those with lower

155

antioxidant intakes. Vitamin E has also been shown to help some diabetics gain better control over their blood sugar.

The new study included 80 overweight adults ages 31 to 65. Overweight and obese individuals have an increased risk of developing insulin resistance, in which the body loses sensitivity to the hormone insulin, causing blood sugar levels to soar.

According to Manning's team, excess fat may speed up the production of oxygen free radicals, the potentially cell-damaging byproducts of normal metabolism. Moreover, overweight people tend to have low levels of antioxidants, which counter the effects of free radicals. It is thought that the resulting oxidative stress may contribute to insulin resistance.

Vitamin K Linked to Lower Diabetes Risk

NEW YORK(Reuters Health) - People who get plenty of vitamin K from food may have a lower risk of developing type 2 diabetes than those who get less of the vitamin, a new study suggests.

Researchers found that among more than 38,000 Dutch adults they followed for a decade, those who got the most vitamin K in their diets were about 20 percent less likely to be diagnosed with type 2 diabetes during the study period.

The findings appear to be the first to show a relationship between vitamin K and diabetes risk, and do not prove that the vitamin is the reason for the lower risk, write the researchers, led by Dr. Joline W.J. Beulens of the University Medical Center Utrecht in the Netherlands.

Instead, they add, the results should fuel further research into whether vitamin K does play a role in the development of type 2 diabetes.

It's estimated that more than 23 million, or nearly 11 percent, of U.S. adults have type 2 diabetes. The most important risk factors for type 2 diabetes include older age, obesity, family history of diabetes and race - - with black, Hispanic and Native Americans at higher risk than whites in the U.S. The extent to which specific nutrients in the diet might affect diabetes risk remains unclear.

Chapter IXV

Vitamin K exists in two natural forms: vitamin K1, or phylloquinone, found largely in green leafy vegetables, as well as some vegetable oils, such as canola and soybean oils; and vitamin K2, or menaquinone, which people get mainly through meat, cheese and eggs.

In the current study, both vitamins K1 and K2 were related to a lower diabetes risk, but the relationship was stronger with vitamin K2.The findings, reported in the journal Diabetes Care, are based on questionnaires from 38,094 men and women who were between the ages of 20 and 70 at the outset. Participants completed a detailed diet survey, from which each person's average vitamin K intake was estimated; they also answered questions on their overall health and lifestyle habits.

Over the next 10 years, 918 study participants were diagnosed with type 2 diabetes, based on their medical records.

In general, Beulens and her colleagues found, the risk of developing type 2 diabetes dipped for every 10-microgram (mcg) increase in vitamin K2 intake. Overall, the one-quarter of participants with the highest intake were 20 percent less likely to be diagnosed with diabetes than the one-quarter with the lowest intake.

With vitamin K1, no decreased risk was seen until consumption of the vitamin was relatively high. Similar to the findings with vitamin K2, the one-quarter of men and women who got the most vitamin K1 were 19 percent less likely to develop diabetes than the quarter with the lowest intake. The researchers accounted for a number of other factors important in diabetes risk, including age, body weight and exercise habits. They also considered other dietary habits, like total calorie intake and consumption of certain other nutrients, like fat, fiber and vitamins C and E.

Still, Higher Vitamin K Intake, Itself, Was Linked to a Lower Diabetes Risk.

Exactly why the vitamin might be protective is not known. However, Beulens and her colleagues note, there is evidence that vitamin K reduces systemic inflammation, which may improve the body's use of the blood-sugar-regulating hormone insulin.

More research, they say, is needed both to confirm these findings and to study the potential underlying reasons.

In the U.S., the recommended daily intake for vitamin K, in all forms, is 120 mcg for men and 90 mcg for women. In this study, participants with the highest intakes typically consumed between 250 and 360 mcg of total vitamin K each day.

Vitamin K Slows Insulin Resistance in Older Men

(HealthDay News) -- Vitamin K slows the development of insulin resistance in older men, but not women, a new study found.

Insulin resistance, a precursor to diabetes, occurs when the body cannot use insulin properly. As a result, glucose builds up in the blood. Overweight and obese people are prone to insulin resistance, because excess fat can interfere with insulin function.

The three-year study, by researchers at the Jean Mayer Human Nutrition Research Center on Aging at Tufts University in Boston, included 355 non-diabetic men and women ages 60 to 80. One group took daily multivitamins containing 500 micrograms of vitamin K (five times the recommended level), along with a calcium and vitamin D supplement. The other (control) group took no vitamin K supplementation but did receive the multivitamin and the calcium and vitamin D supplement. Both groups were told to keep eating their normal diets.

By the end of the study, the men who took vitamin K had improved insulin resistance and lower blood insulin levels than men in the control group. The study was published in the November issue of the journal Diabetes Care.

The amount of vitamin K contained in the supplements used in the study is attainable by consuming a healthy diet, the researchers said. Brussels sprouts, broccoli, and dark, leafy greens (such as spinach and collards) are good sources of vitamin K.

For More information see: Tufts University, news release, Nov. 26, 2008

Chapter IXV

FOODS FOR DIABETES

AlMOND AND DIABETES: Researchers have found that eating more almonds helps prevent type 2 diabetes and heart disease. It does so by improving your insulin sensitivity and lowering levels of LDL ("bad") cholesterol. A new study has found that almonds are one way to improve your insulin sensitivity and lower LDL ("bad") cholesterol in people with prediabetes. Researchers looked at the effects of consuming an almond- enriched diet on factors linked to the progression of type 2 diabetes and heart disease. It included 65 adults with prediabetes, average age 54. They either received a control diet (15%-20% calories from protein, 10% total energy from saturated fat, 60%-70% from carbohydrate and monounsaturated fatty acids and cholesterol) or a diet that ensured that 20% of the calories came from almonds. The study lasted four months. Those people eating almonds showed significantly improved LDL-cholesterol levels and measures of insulin sensitivity. Both are huge risk factors for heart disease and type 2 diabetes.

Nutrients in almonds, such as fiber and unsaturated fat, have been shown to help reduce LDL-cholesterol levels, increase insulin sensitivity and increase beta-cell function, all of which can help to prevent the development of type 2 diabetes and reduce the risk of cardiovascular disease. These explain why the almond group in the study experienced such health benefits.

APPLE CIDER VINEGAR AND DIABETES

A daily tonic of apple cider vinegar (2 or 3 teaspoons to 8 ounces of water) supplies dietary fiber and other ingredients, which are beneficial in controlling blood glucose levels. As well, the acids and enzymes promote better digestion and nutrient absorption, which is impaired in many diabetes sufferers.

This home remedy has been the subject of new research that shows that apple cider vinegar can help lower blood sugar levels hence it is highly recommended to be used with green salads and sunflower oil on daily basis.

Bairley Beta Glucan

Powerful Benefits of Barley's Beta-Glucan for Diabetes

(HealthCastle.com) You may already know that barley is a health food that helps lower cholesterol. So, you probably won't be surprised to learn that studies have shown this whole-grain barley helps lower LDL cholesterol, the bad kind of cholesterol. In 2005, the FDA approved the coronary heart disease risk reduction health claim for beta-glucan found in barley.

Beta-Glucan and Diabetes: Beta-glucan is a type of soluble fiber. Findings from clinical trials showed that people who ate foods containing barley experienced significant reductions in glucose compared to responses after eating similar products with similar glycemic index (GI) containing other resistant starch. Another small study published in 2007 in the Diabetes Research and Clinical Practice Journal reported a 30% decrease in Hemoglobin A1C (HbA1c) - from 8.4% to 5.9% - in people with type 2 diabetes who ate a healthy diet including pearl barley that supplied 18 grams of soluble fiber per day. This is a significant drop, as the American Diabetes Association's recommended target for HbA1c is 7%.

Researchers at the Creighton Diabetes Center in Nebraska found that when people ate a breakfast cereal made from fiber-rich barley, their blood sugar remained 600% lower than when they ate oatmeal -- which is thought to be one of the best "slow carbs" you can eat. Reason? Barley is high in a particular type of fiber called beta-glucan that's super-effective at slowing the conversion of carbs to glucose.

Other Food Sources Containing Beta-Glucan are: Shiitake mushroom,Peas, Beans,Oats, Yeast...

Budwig Diet For Diabetics: Details of the Cure

NOTE: Each time you make a batch of the Budwig Diet, consume it within 10 minutes so it does not deteriorate in potency. Also, do not add anything into the mixture until AFTER the cottage cheese and flax seed oil have completely mixed together. Because the Budwig Diet Mixture is used for multiple diseases, a separate article has been written on how to make the Budwig Diet Mixture

Chapter IXV

How to Make the Budwig Mixture

A diabetic should take at least <u>4 tablespoons</u> of the flaxseed oil every day as part of their treatment. That is the minimum dose.

You can make one mixture twice a day or you can make one very large mixture once a day. It doesn't matter. Remember to shake the bottle of flaxseed oil each time before you use it and remember to eat the mixture within half an hour after making it.

Also, do **NOT** use flax seeds or flaxseed cereal as part of the mixture (but they can be added after it is mixed). The whole point to making the Budwig mixture is to convert oil soluble omega-3 into water soluble omega-3 and this can only be done with oils.

When buying fish oils it is critical to make sure the oils do not have mercury and other heavy metals in it. That is why I endorse the high quality Norwegian products.

Take Omega-3 Fatty Acids to Reduce Inflammation.These healthy fats improve the body's ability to respond to insulin, reduce inflammation, lower blood lipids and prevent excessive blood clotting. Good dietary sources of omega-3 fatty acids include cold-water fish, such as salmon or cod (eat two or three times a week), olive or canola oil, flaxseed and English walnuts.

CAMEL MILK: is a miracle gift from GOD, and it is a must for all diseases including diabetes and its consequences(for more details read Chapter 14 of this book)

CAMEL URINE WONDERS FOR DIABETES:

A number of researchers in Saudi Arabia, India and Kenya arrived at miracle results by using camel urine for different cases of cancer, liver cirrhosis, diabetes,hypertension, SLE, auto-immune diseases.

Chamomile Tea: Drinking chamomile tea, a rich source of antioxidants, may help prevent diabetes complications, such as blindness, nerve damage and kidney problems, say UK and Japanese scientists. In a trial of diabetic rats, those fed chamomile experienced a decrease in blood glucose levels associated with induced stress, leading to fewer degenerative changes in tissue associated with inflammation. These findings were reported online in the August 6, 2008, issue of Journal of Agricultural and Food Chemistry.

Chlorella: Lowers Cholesterol, Body Fat and Blood Sugar (Superfood update)

If you are interested in reducing body fat, getting your cholesterol level under control and staying clear of diabetes, chlorella may be just the perfect superfood. Researchers have recently investigated the effects of Chlorella on people with high-risk factors for lifestyle diseases and found that chlorella affects a positive outcome by controlling gene expression. Other new findings have also added to chlorella's impressive credentials.

As reported in the September edition of the *Journal of Medicinal Food*, researchers in Kyoto, chlorella intake resulted in noticeable reductions in body fat percentages, total serum cholesterol, and fasting blood glucose levels.

Chlorella reduces UVB degradation of the skin

The May-June edition of the *European Journal of Dermatology* reports that solar UV radiation damages human skin, affects skin tone and resiliency, and leads to premature aging. Skin damage by oxidants leads to activation of protein kinase C, increasing collagen degradation. Ingestion of chlorella has been shown to inhibit this activity.

Chlorella decreases dioxin and increases immunoglobulin concentration in breast milk

One of the big sales pitches for the use of infant formula in place of breast milk has been that breast milk contains dangerous levels of dioxin. A study reported in the March, 2007 edition of the *Journal of Medicinal Food* analyzed dioxin levels in breast milk and maternal blood samples from 35 pregnant women in Japan. The researchers found that toxic equivalents were significantly lower in the breast milk of the women taking chlorella tablets than in the control group. These results suggest that chlorella supplementation by the mother may reduce transfer of dioxins to the child through the breast milk.

New studies also document the powerful chelating properties of chlorella

Chapter IXV

Also reported in the September *Journal of Medicinal Food* is a study in which 40 rats were divided into one control group and three groups that were treated with cadmium. One cadmium group received no chlorella, one received 5% chlorella, and one received 10% chlorella. After 8 weeks, the relative liver weight was significantly lower in the group receiving no chlorella compared with both groups receiving chlorella, indicating severe liver damage in the no-chlorella group. This group also displayed significantly higher hepatic concentrations of cadmium than the groups receiving chlorella. Hepatic RNA had a higher expression in the chlorella treated groups than in the no-chlorella group. Researchers concluded that chlorella has a protective effect against cadmium induced lever damage by reducing cadmium accumulation and stimulating the expression of RNA in the liver.

The July edition of *Food Chemistry Toxicology* reports another study in which the chelating ability of chlorella was assessed. Monitoring of lead poisoning demonstrated that chlorella treatment significantly reduced lead levels in blood and tissues, completely restored the normal levels of ALA in the liver, and decreased the abnormally high plasma levels of ALA.

The findings of these two studies underscore the powerful chelating ability of chlorella and suggest that chlorella would be useful for pre-treating before consuming any food or drink in which the presence of heavy metals is suspected, such as fish. Chlorella has also been shown in previous studies to be an effective chelator of mercury and is an excellent supplement for anyone with dental fillings containing mercury, as well as anyone undergoing the removal of fillings.

What is chlorella?

Chlorella is tiny, single-celled water-grown green algae that contain a nucleus and an enormous amount of readily available chlorophyll. It is composed of about 58% highly digestible protein, and carbohydrates. It is a good dietary choice for people who do not eat meat. It contains all of the B vitamins, vitamins C and E, amino acids, beta-carotene, iron, zinc, macro-minerals such as calcium, magnesium, zinc, potassium, rare trace minerals, essential fatty acids including GLA, and polysaccharides. One teaspoon of chlorella contains 90 mg of RNA and 8 mg of DNA.

Chlorella has more vitamin B-12 than liver. It is virtually a complete food and considered one of the superfoods, delivering a wind fall of nutrition to the body.

Chlorella contains thousands of phytochemicals, most of which have not yet been identified.chlorella is nature's answer to the multi-vitamin pill concept, offering a broad array of nutrients in highly bio-available form with perfect synergy. It has shown to be effective at reversing degenerative diseases such as all types of cancers, diabetes, liver disorders, high blood pressure, and obesity.

People with poor digestion are able to easily digest chlorella. Chlorella has been shown to accelerate healing, protect against radiation, help in the treatment of Candida albicans and relieve arthritis pain. It is effective against anemia and its stimulation of red blood cells assures proper transport of oxygen to the brain and body.

Chlorella is a potent cancer fighter

Chlorella stimulates the immune system and the production of interferon, one of the body's greatest natural defenses against cancer. Increased interferon production is thought to stimulate macrophages, T-cells and tumor necrosis factor. This results in the immune system being able to combat foreign invaders whether they are viruses, bacteria, chemicals or foreign proteins. Chlorella's DNA repair mechanism has been documented.

Numerous animal studies have documented chlorella's effectiveness against cancer. One such study involved mice given chlorella prior to being transplanted with breast tumors. The results indicated a 70 percent survival rate in the chlorella fed group and a control group survival rate of zero.

In another study, fifteen glioblastoma patients were treated with high levels of chlorella, in some cases combined with chemotherapy and radiation. Glioblastoma is the type of deadly brain tumor recently diagnosed in Senator Kennedy. Their health and immune status increased immediately, and they experienced a 40 percent two-year survival rate, compared to the normal two year survival rate of 10 percent for this type of cancer.

Chapter IXV

Chlorella helps balance the body's pH

It is believed by many that disease starts and thrives in an acidic body environment. Any diet that is deficient in fruits and vegetables will be acidic in nature. The consumption of soft drinks and processed fruit drinks are particularly acid forming as are diets high in meat and uncultured dairy products.Proper pH balance is critical for health, and the body goes to great lengths to maintain the proper pH of its blood, by increasing respiration and by pulling alkaline minerals out of the bones to use to buffer any excess acidity. This is why consumption of soft drinks is linked to osteoporosis.

Chlorella is an alkaline food, which means it counters acidity. This promotes increased bone mass since the body is not sacrificing minerals from the bones to create proper acid/alkaline balance. Metabolic function is therefore improved. The consumption of alkaline foods has been linked to improved immune function, kidney function, higher energy levels, and lower allergic response levels.

Coconut Oil Benefits Blood Sugar and Fights Diabetes

Bruce Fife explains how coconut oil slows down the absorption of sugar in the blood stream and helps the pancreas with improving insulin sensitivity, which is very beneficial to diabetics. He discusses the ability of coconut oil to improve circulation and it's benefits in fighting and reversing the numbness in the legs and feet that many people with diabetes experience.

Coconut oil diabetes benefits allow your *cells* to feed even without the aid of *insulin*. Coconut oil *(CNO)* may be one of the best foods for *diabetics*. Let me explain.

Insulin is crucial because without it, fatty acids and glucose in the blood stream won't be able to enter and feed your cells. *Mitochondria*, the energy producing organs of cells, transform glucose and fatty acids into *fuel* to power metabolic functions and for cell nourishment.Glucose and *long chain fatty acids (LCFA)* have one big problem. They cannot enter your cells without insulin. *Medium chain fatty acids (MCFA)* richly and uniquely found in coconut oil can penetrate the mitochondria's double membrane without the assistance of the hormone insulin.

165

It doesn't matter whether your *pancreas* is producing enough insulin or your cells are *insulin-resistant*. You can rest assured that MCFA-rich coconut oil can still nourish your cells. What a comforting diabetic fact.

Because MCFAs can keep cells nourished, capillaries and blood vessels are kept alive and healthy which helps you a lot in preventing the development of atherosclerosis. At this point, it should be clear that coconut oil improves the *circulation* and *cardiovascular health* of diabetics. Coconut oil does not block arteries. It even opens them up. In addition to its ability to feed your all important cells without the need for insulin, MCFAs abundantly found in coconut oil also help improve *insulin secretion, insulin sensitivity* and *glucose tolerance*. MCFAs stimulate metabolism which increases insulin production and glucose absorption into your cells. For this reason, coconut oil can help many diabetics reduce their dependency on insulin medication.

Coconut oil can also help regulate your *blood sugar* levels. It slows down the emptying of the stomach so that sugars are released at a slower rate into the bloodstream. Coconut oil has a very low *glycemic index* which is a system of measuring the effect of specific foods on blood sugar.Even the glycemic index of sweets and starchy foods are substantially lowered when coconut oil is added to them. Adding the versatile coconut oil to meals is very effective in lowering the glycemic index of your favorite foods.

Coconut oil diabetes blessings help address the underlying problem right at the cellular level. Do you now see why coconut oil may be one of the healthiest foods in the fight against diabetes?

COFFEE AND DIABETES

Is caffeine behind coffee's anti-diabetic effects?

Stephen Daniells, wrote on 10-Jun-2010: Coffee's widely-reported potential anti-diabetes benefits may be related to the caffeine content of the beverage, claims a new study from Japan.

Scientists from Nagoya University report that coffeeprevented the development of high-blood sugar in lab mice, as well as improving their sensitivity to insulin, thereby reducing the risk of diabetes.

Chapter IXV

"Our results indicated that caffeine is one of the most effective anti-diabetic compounds in coffee," wrote the researchers in the Journal of Agricultural and Food Chemistry.

"We hope to identify the target tissues upon which coffee or caffeine acts directly, as well as effective anti-diabetic compounds other than caffeine. However, the present results suggest that coffee consumption may help to prevent type-2 diabetes and metabolic syndrome," they added. The results are consistent with a growing body of research, much of which was pulled together in a meta-analysis in the Archives of Internal Medicine(Dec 2009, Vol. 169, pp. 2053-2063) by scientists from the University of Sydney, Australia. Data from over 500,000 individuals with over 21,000 cases of type-2 diabetes from prospective studies showed that drinking three to four coffee and tea may reduce the risk of developing diabetes by 25 percent.

Benefits of the coffee bean : Coffee, one of the world's largest traded commodities produced in more than 60 countries and generating more than $70bn in retail sales a year, continues to spawn research and interest with data linking it to improved liver health, in addition to the potential anti-diabetes benefits.

Diabetes affects an estimated 24 million Americans, equal to 8 percent of the population. The total costs are thought to be as much as $174 billion, with $116 billion being direct costs from medication, according to 2005-2007 American Diabetes Association figures.

Cucumber for Diabetes

Anti-diabetic Benefits of Cucumber:

Beta cells present in the pancreas produce the hormone insulin.Cucumber is found to possess a hormone required by the beta cells in the insulin production.Moreover, the Glycemic Index of cumcuber is found to be zero.Every food item contains essential nutrients in varied proportions.The presence of the nutrient carbohydrate and its effect on the body is measured by the quantity Glycemic Index.The carbohydrates are primarily responsible for raise in the glucose level.But the carbohydrates present in the cucumber is easily digestible in a diabetes patient's stomach.That is why,the Glycemic Index of this vegetable is Zero.This

167

keeps the glucose level after the intake of this vegetable in check. A Supplement called Spiny Sea Cucumber Extract Powder is found to be effective in combating Diabetes.

Eggplant for Type 2 Diabetes: The National Diabetes Education Program, Mayo Clinic and American Diabetes Association recommend an eggplant based diet as a choice for management of **type 2 diabetes.** The rationale for this suggestion is the high fiber and low soluble carbohydrate content of eggplant.

Study results indicate that phenolic-enriched extracts of eggplant inhibit enzymes that provide a strong biochemical basis for management of type 2 diabetes by controlling glucose absorption and reducing associated high blood pressure (hypertension).

It also reduce cholesterol and new studies show it is useful for cancer and high blood pressure.

Fish Twice a Week Cuts Diabetics' Kidney Risks

Dietary change enhances blood glucose control, study finds

(HealthDay News) -- Eating fish twice a week may help reduce the risk of kidney disease in people with diabetes, according to a British study of more than 22,000 adults, including 517 with diabetes. The study was published in the November issue of the American Journal of Kidney Diseases. In addition to eating fish, other measures that help lower the risk of albuminuria include tight control of glucose, keeping blood pressure under control, quitting smoking, and following a diabetic diet as prescribed by a doctor, according to the kidney foundation.

Fresh Ginger Juice : Drinking fresh ginger juice has worked wonders for persons with diabetes. You have to be careful not to drink too much as it can lower your blood sugar levels too severely. Results have been reported to be all but instantaneous. Juice a very small amount, and mix with water.

Flaxseed Oil: Take two tablespoons of high quality flaxseed oil daily. You will notice within a few weeks that your blood sugar levels will drop.

Chapter IXV

GRAPEFRUIT MAY CURE DIABETES

The Daily Mirrortoday hails grapefruit as a "fruity 'cure' for diabetes". The newspaper suggests that the chemical naringenin found in the fruit "can do the same job as two drugs used to treat type-2 diabetes".

Surprisingly, the research in question only looked at the effects of naringenin on human and rat liver cells in the laboratory. This very preliminary research has certainly not identified a "cure" for diabetes.

The study was carried out by researchers from Shriners Hospitals in Boston and other research centres in the US, Israel and France. This study was covered by the Daily Mirror, Daily Mail and Daily Express. All of these newspapers claim that grapefruit can "fight" or "cure" diabetes, and that it has the same benefits as two diabetes drugs. These claims wildly over-extrapolate the findings of this preliminary laboratory research. None of the newspaper reports clarify that this was only laboratory research on isolated cells or that any potential benefits or side effects of naringenin will remain unclear until there are human studies.

Finally, the researchers found that treating freshly extracted rat liver cells with naringenin for 24 hours reduced their production of a type of fat called triglycerides, and also reduced their production of bile salts.

Conclusion: This complex laboratory research suggests that naringenin can affect proteins and genes involved in fat metabolism in liver cells. Although the effect that it has on the cells is similar to the effects of drugs such as the fibrates and glitazones, this does not necessarily mean that naringenin could be used to treat the

Green Beans: are traditionally known to lower blood sugar levels in even those with type 1 diabetes. Eat them fresh and often.

Indian Gooseberry: with its high vitamin C content, is considered valuable in diabetes. A tablespoon of its juice, mixed with a cup of bitter gourd juice, taken daily for two months, will stimulate the islets of Langerhans, that is, the isolated group of cells that secrete the hormone insulin in the pancreas. This mixture reduces the blood sugar in diabetes.

KIWI FRUIT FOR DIABETES

Fights Diseases & Lowers Blood Sugar and Cholesterol

Kiwifruits are high in fiber, making them good for digestion. Fruits that are high in fiber help to improve diseases like diabetes. A natural occurring sugar alcohol, called inositol, is present in the kiwi. This compound might have a positive effect in the regulation of diabetes. This compound might also help with nerve conduction velocity, which is found in diabetic neuropathy.

Fiber helps to control sugar levels, and binds to toxic substances located in the colon. This helps to eliminate the toxic compounds from the colon which makes the organ function better. Diets high in fiber have also been proven to lower cholesterol levels, improve the health of people suffering from cardiovascular diseases, and lower the risk of a heart attack. One of the aspects for a healthy heart is an adequate sodium to potassium ratio. This ratio is excellent in the kiwifruit. This aspect lessens the chance that a person will have hypertension.

Good For Your Eyes

The kiwifruit contains high amounts of vitamins A, C, and E which are the most typical anti-oxidant vitamins. The Archives of Ophthalmology have published a series of studies that has proven that eating three servings or more of fruit can lessen the risk of developing macular degeneration, which is an age related eye disease. The study was performed on 110,000 men and women that took place over several decades. The study showed that the people who ate fruits containing a high amount of vitamins A, C, and E had a better protection rate against macular degeneration than those who ate fewer of these fruits.

Fights Aging

Along with protecting against macular degeneration, the vitamins A, C, and E are very powerful in helping to fight off signs of aging. The high amounts of these vitamins in the kiwifruit have been proven to fight off damage done by free radicals. Free radicals can destroy the cells in the body and cause early aging signs as well as various diseases, such as cancer and cardiovascular disease.

Chapter IXV

Contains Minerals

Another great benefit of the kiwifruit is the fact that it is loaded with a variety of minerals, or electrolytes, that are necessary for the replenishment of these electrolytes during exercise. This electrolyte replenishment is especially important for people who live in a hot environment. The Chinese came up with a kiwi-based sports drink that was designed particularly to help boost electrolytes in athletes that trained in hot environments. They added a 5% increase of carbohydrates to this juice to help regulate and maintain glucose levels while the athletes were training.

Aids in Weight Loss

A **weight loss fruit**, the kiwifruit is an excellent fruit to eat when losing weight. One kiwi contains just 45 calories, 3 grams of fat, 1 gram of protein, 11 grams of carbohydrates, and 2.5 grams of fiber. This is one of the fruits that are lowest in calories. The fiber in the kiwi will help you feel fuller longer, and there's no harm at all in eating more that one at a time. Kiwifruits are also high in potassium, in fact, they have the same amount as bananas. Potassium is great for sore muscle relief.

Lettuce and Diabetes : Diabetes Cure Could Come From Lettuce, Researchers Say

Florida Lab Has Success Injecting Lettuce With Human Gene For Insulin

A researcher at the University of Central Florida says he has created a strain of lettuce that actually creates insulin. For people with diabetes, it could mean the end of insulin injections -- and the folks in the lab say it could even be a cure for diabetes.

For the last five years, lettuce has ruled Dr. Henry Daniell's life.

Genetically-modified lettuce is being grown in a lab at UCF. A leaf is placed in a machine and then injected with the human gene for insulin, Daniell said. Daniell first tested his insulin-producing lettuce on mice. He said by the end of the study, the diabetic mice had normal blood and urine sugar levels and their cells were producing normal levels of insulin after eight weeks of treatment.

171

Human trials are now under way. Researchers said that the lettuce can be ground to a fine, green powder to be used in the form of capsules.

According to Daniell, the treatment can not only prevent diabetes before symptoms appear, but it can also treat the disease in later stages. The researchers believe that if this insulin-loaded lettuce works as well on people as it does in mice, treatment for diabetes could take only a few weeks, and then it's impossible to know just how important this could become for the central coast and all of California's lettuce growers.

Milk Thistle, (Silymarin): The extract from seeds of the Milk Thistle, Silybum marianum (silymarin) is known to have antioxidant properties. Research shows that this extract can help people significantly lower the amount of sugar bound to haemoglobin in blood, as well as reducing fasting blood sugar levels. Silymarin contains a number of active constituents called flavolignans which are also used to help protect the liver from poisoning.

Noni Juice: is very helpful for diabetes and many former diabetics have credited it for curing their diabetes.

Okra: Infuse 2-3 fingers of okra overnight and drink its water in the morning and notice the difference in blood sugar reading.

Parslane: The seeds of parslane are useful in diabetes. A teaspoon of the seeds should be taken every day with half a cup of water . They increase the body's own insulin and help in curing diabetes.

Sage Tea: is a very old and well known herb to help lower and maintain a stable blood sugar level by diabetics. Simply use tea bags or steep the leaves.

RED PEPPER AND DIABETES

Here is another Diabetic Life Diet food discovery that came about partly by accident.It seems odd to us now that we didn't learn about this or read about it before we discovered it through our own blood glucose monitoring, but I think that is how food discovery works for most diabetics. Each and every diabetic responds uniquely to foods on account of the complexity of the root causes of diabetes, so it makes it very hard to know what will work for you - even if it is reported to work for others.

Chapter IXV

You may find that a food or combination of food is fine for you to eat, but is not for a friend or relative. In my case, my father is also a type 2 diabetic, and what he can eat is not the same as what I can eat.

The most important thing is to not be discouraged if you hear that some particular food is a wonderful food for blood glucose control, but it doesn't work for you. I'll detail my own discoveries along this line - as I have had plenty.

We've periodically cooked with dried chili peppers as part of our regular meals for many many years just because we like to mix it up sometimes for the hot peppers taste and fun of it. Not too long ago we started to use dried chili peppers again. As for our path to discover the diabetes pitaya fruit link, in our regular monitoring of our blood sugar levels after meals we noticed a reduction in our post meal blood glucose levels and in our fasting blood glucose levels.

The only real change we had been making was using the dried chili peppers, and that led us to do some research on what might be happening. It turns out that there are plenty of references (once you know to look) to the possible health benefits of capsaicin diabetes control. That led me to further optimize my source of capsaicin from the dried chili peppers (which sometimes have lost their potency, and which require the use of more oil than you may like in cooking - as well as the requirement to heat the oil which degrades the health benefits of healthy oils like olive oil or canola oil).

Now I know that hot chile pepper diabetes controls a great benefit of eating hot peppers as part of my diabetic diet plan. If like me you tolerate and hopefully enjoy hot chile peppers diabetes benefits are easy and immediate. See if you start to realize the benefits of capsaicin diabetes control by including hot peppers like habano peppers in your diabetic die trecipes. For me, habanero peppers diabetes control yields the most benefits towards lowering blood glucose levels including next day fasting blood glucose levels because habano peppers are some of the very hottest peppers and have more capsaicin. More capsaicin means greater capsaicin diabetes control. Serranno peppers are about one tenth as hot as habano peppers, and have about one tenth the habanero peppers diabetes control effects for that reason. Hot chile peppers diabetes benefits and

173

overall benefits of hot peppers diabetes control are substantial for me - and I hope they will be the same for you.

I can't say this is a capsaicin diabetes cure, but the health benefits of capsaicin diabetes control for me go a long way toward making my type 2 diabetes easier to manage.

Yellow Dock Tea: How be it little known, yellow dock tea works wonders for diabetics. Steady use has been reported to eliminate even severe diabetic symptoms.

YOGURT FOR DIABETES

Yogurt is a Diabetes Healing Superfood because of the importance of probiotics for proper glucose digestion and metabolism. However, not all yogurts are equal. Many store-bought products can be loaded with sugar, artificial flavors and additives that are not good for you. To be sure you get the best healing micro-organisms in your yogurt, it's best to make your own at home.

Researchers have uncovered a substance in dairy fat that could drastically drop your risk of ever developing Type II diabetes. The fatty acid—called trans-palmitoleic acid—cannot be produced by your body. So the only way you can get it is by eating dairy or meat products.

The study...conducted by researchers at the Harvard School of Public Health...examined the data from the participants in the 20-year-long Cardiovascular Health Study funded by the National Heart, Lung, and Blood Institute. It was found that those volunteers with higher levels of trans-palmitoleic acid had healthier blood-cholesterol levels, less inflammation, and more controlled insulin levels.

In addition, those with the highest level of the acid circulating in their blood were 60% less likely to develop diabetes as compared with those participants with the lowest levels of the compound.

Wheat Germ Oil : A strong source of fiber, which benefits digestion, but also proves beneficial to patients with diabetes since fiber doesn't raise glucose levels.

Wheat Germ strengthens the immune system,It balances metabolism and improves oxygen use within the body, improves skin and helps in the

Chapter IXV

repair of tissues, helps increase stamina and the storage of muscle energy, lowers cholesterol levels and protects heart, and It is good for weight loss.

Foods to avoid

It is always advisable to avoid some foods if you are diabetic such as refined sugar, sweets, syrups, glucose, jam, molasses, fruit sugar, ice-cream, cakes, pastries, sweet biscuits, chocolates, soft drinks, condensed milk, cream and fried foods. Fats like butter, ghee and hydrogenated vegetable oil should also be avoided. White sugar and white flour should be reduced drastically. Avoid all processed foods, junk food, pastries, cookies, canned and preserved foods. They contain harmful preservatives and lot of salt. Avoid soft drinks since these have a lot of sugar. Try to avoid fried foods from your diet.

Smoking results in the using up of oxygen in the body. It will result in less of oxygen needed by the body to metabolize glucose. So smoking should be avoided.

Foods to be limited

Salt consumption should be reduced to a minimum. You will get enough salt form the vegetables and fruits you eat. Reduce animal foods especially red meats. Reduce poultry and egg. Reduce caffeine and alcohol. Do not drink tea and coffee more than 2 cups a day. Try to replace it with green tea or herbal teas like Parsley tea, Blueberry leaf, Tea made of tender walnut tree leaves, Water in which kidney bean pods have been cooked is good diabetes.

Do not consume alcohol in empty stomach. Alcohol on an empty stomach can cause low blood glucose or hypoglycemia.Foods that should be consumed in moderation are honey and other natural sugars like palm sugar, dates which can be used instead of white sugar. Remember these should be consumed in very little quantity only.Pasta, coconut, other nuts, unsweetened juices, eggs should be limited. You can replace it with whole grain, unpolished rice and Soya products. Try to eat whole grain bread instead of white flour. Fats like olive oil and peanut oil are more advisable that hydrogenated fats. Low fat food like skimmed milk and low fat home made cottage cheese can be taken in moderation. You can

175

also substitute it with yoghurt. Sea food and fish also can be taken in moderation.

Foods to be taken

Drink at least 8 glasses of water a day. An alkaline diet with natural food is recommended. Wholegrain, fruits, nuts, vegetables, and dairy products form a good diet for the diabetic. Raw vegetables can be taken in high quantities. It has been found that cooked foods raise blood glucose higher than raw, unpeeled foods. Cooking destroys many of the enzymes and some vitamins and minerals.

Eat at least five fruits every day. Fruits like grape fruit, pomegranate juice, Indian blackberry, banana, granny smith apples, fig, cranberries, black berry, kiwi fruits, and citrus fruits are highly recommended. It can be taken as a snack. Cucumber, Lettuce, onion, garlic string beans cucumber radish, tomato, carrot, leaves; spinach turnip, cabbage and Jerusalem artichoke are good for diabetes. Colorful vegetables are good for the functioning of pancreas. Drink Fruit juices without sugar. Brewer's yeast and sprouted alfalfa and mung beans are good for the body. Unripe banana also can be cooked and eaten.

The most important of all is eating high fiber diet which lowers need for insulin. It releases energy into the body slowly. It has also been found that diabetes decreases and may even disappear in people eating a high fiber or whole food diet. High fiber diet has more chromium and chromium is very good for people with diabetes.

Eat lot of potassium rich foods like raw peanuts, tomato, bananas, melons, dried peas, potatoes, apple cider vinegar, skimmed milk powder, wheat but do not take potassium supplements.Include soluble fiber in your meals like barley, oatmeal, almond meal, dried beans, kidney beans, cooked black beans, peas, cereals, chickpeas, Bengal gram which has low glycemic index, , Black gram, lentils and corn or garbanzo beans to helps considerably in reducing blood sugar levels. Soy products like tofu, tempeh, soymilk, soya powder, soy bean sprouts, nuggets etc are also very good in containing neurological complications in diabetes. You can make bread out of any of the whole grains. Get a lot of soluble fiber into your diet. When you eat lots of bread, cereal and starchy vegetables you will get enough of starches which is very helpful for diabetes. Insoluble

Chapter IXV

fibers, found in bran (oat bran, wheat bran), whole grain breads, whole grains and nuts, act as intestinal scrubbers by cleaning out the lower gastrointestinal tract. Fiber cleans your intestinal tract by moving out the food so that it wouldn't stay there and putrefy. Butter milk and yoghurt diet are very beneficial.

Magnesium supplementation has been shown to improve insulin sensitivity. Chromium: Whole grains, seeds, mushrooms, corn oil and brewer's yeast are relatively good sources of biologically valuable chromium.

MINERALS FOR DIABETES

CALCIUM & MAGNESIUM AND DIABETES:

Numerous studies suggest that calcium, magnesium and potassium are essential minerals that promote good health including healthy cardiovascular function, bone health and favorable blood pressure. Along with a multi-vitamin, I recommend consuming 3,500 mg per day of potassium, 1,000 mg per day of calcium (500 mg if you take calcium citrate malate, which has superior absorption) and 500 mg per day of magnesium.

A study focused on 64,000 women (with no elevated blood sugar or other chronic health concerns2) found that women with the highest intake of calcium and magnesium had a statistically decreased incidence of later developing elevated blood sugar. The researchers' data suggests that the combined intake of calcium and magnesium may protect against the development of elevated blood sugar.

(Please see: Villegas R, Gao YT, Dai Q, et al., Dietary calcium and magnesium intakes and the risk of type 2 diabetes: the Shanghai Women's Health Study, The American Journal of Clinical Nutrition. April 2009, Pp 1059-1067).

CHROMIUM :Chromium Picolinate and Polynicotinate improve the ability of insulin to lower blood sugar levels. If you are diabetic, consult your doctor before taking chromium.

To Prevent Diabetes....... Chromium to Normalize Sugar Levels

177

Dr. Mansour

Your body requires adequate levels of chromium to properly control blood glucose levels. This essential trace mineral aids in the uptake of blood sugar into the body's cells, where it can be used to generate energy more efficiently. It's also helpful in reducing sweet cravings.

Chromium: is an excellent supplement to take for helping the body use sugar more efficiently. Chromium helps cells to respond better to naturally producing insulin. Some rich sources of chromium are seeds and whole grains. Also mushrooms.

GTF Chromium (Glucose Transport Factor Chromium) - The primary role of insulin is glucose transport is the primary role of insulin, chromium's main function is increasing insulin's efficiency in regulating blood sugar levels. In one study of 180 men and women with Type II diabetes, researchers divided the subjects into three groups, each receiving twice daily doses of either 200 mcg or 500 mcg of chromium or a placebo. The patients were allowed to continue with their usual diet and medications. At the end of two months, those who took 1,000 mcg of chromium daily showed significant improvement in insulin response, the number if insulin receptors, and levels of blood lipids (fats and cholesterol)0. It took four months the group taking 400 mcg chromium daily to improve as much as the higher dosage group. However, all the patients taking chromium showed measurable improvement in their diabetes-related symptoms: It Helps Insulin health , Increases energy ,Lowers lipid levels ,Promotes weight loss and Improves body composition

Brewers Yeast is rich in chromium and hence it is recommended for diabetics

VANADIUM: assists insulin in metabolizing glucose. The human studies with Vanadium executed so far are impressive: they show that it can greatly reduce the needs for insulin and hypoglycemic medications. Vanadium also lowers blood sugar as well as the need for insulin. Vanadyl sulfate has been found to benefit both Type I and Type II diabetes. In humans it appears to have the insulin-mimicking effect that Type I diabetics need, as well as the ability to overcome the insulin resistance that is the defining abnormality in Type II diabetes.

178

Chapter IXV

ZINC: has shown to be deficient in diabetic patients. Zinc is best absorbed as lozenges.

Zinc: is essential for the pancreas to produce insulin and makes insulin work effectively. It also helps in fortifying the insulin receptor cells. When zinc is low, the pancreas does not create sufficient insulin, thus high glucose levels .Zinc is an immunity booster, used for colds,flu and infections.It is essential for men sexual health ,infertility for men and women.It enhances testosterone   for sex and diabetes,and prevents prostate enlargement.

OTHER DIETARY SUPPLEMENTS:

ALPHA LIOPIC ACID: is used for the treatment of nerve damage and helps control blood sugar levels.Alpha Lipoic Acid - In Germany, alpha-lipoic acid is an approved medical treatment for peripheral neuropathy, a common complication of diabetes. It speeds the removal of glucose from the bloodstream, at least partly by enhancing insulin function, and it reduces insulin resistance, an underpinning of many cases of coronary heart disease and obesity. The therapeutic dose for lipoic acid is 600 mg/day. In the United States, it is sold as a dietary supplement, usually as 50 mg tablets. (The richest food source of alpha-lipoic acid is red meat – but to insure proper health, use lean cuts of organic beef that has not been subject to antibiotics or feed lot practices).

In accordance with FDA regulation, we do not make any therapeutic claims for any Dietary Supplements in accordance with the Dietary Supplement Health and Education Act. Alpha-Lipoic Acid: helps to reduce the bodies blood sugars. It allows the cells to utilize energy more efficiently which is very beneficial for diabetics, and has been seen to lower their blood sugar count by more than 30, single handedly.

Boost Antioxidant Levels with Alpha-Lipoic Acid

This powerful antioxidant kills free radicals that damage cells and cause pain, inflammation, burning, tingling and numbness in people who have peripheral neuropathy (nerve damage) caused by diabetes. Studies also suggest that alpha-lipoic acid (ALA) enables the body to utilize glucose more efficiently. It helps for diabetes, cholesterol,heart,brain,eye disorders and and as an excellent antioxidant.

I need to mention some comments from the superb book: **The pH Miracle for Diabetes**, by the brilliant researcher Dr. Robert O. Young, PhD. On page 84 he mentions that the body converts alpha lipoic acid into forms of omega-3. On page 111 he recommends a ratio of omega-3 to omega-6 of 3:1 and he recommends borage oil (1,000 mg capsule three times a day) to get the omega-6 GLA (gamma-linolenic acid), LA (linoleic acid) and EA (erucic acid). That is good advice.

BIOTIN: Biotin plays an important role in energy metabolism,fat and glycogen synthesis,breaking down carbohydrates, and weight loss.

COENZYME Q10(CQ10) AND DIABETES

Did you know that the vitamin-like substance, Coenzyme Q10, reduces your blood glucose by 30 percent and stimulates insulin production in your body? Read more about natural remedies like this one in your copy of Forbidden Secrets From Nature's Pharmacy. Go here to order.

Glutathione - Aids in breaking down glucose into energy,and works as an antioxidant against inflammation which is a major cause of type 2 diabetes according to researchers in the Medical College at the University of Clifornia at St. Diego.

L-Carnitine, L-Glutamine and Taurine help mobilize fat, reduce sugar cravings and assist the release of insulin.

Quercetin helps protect the membranes of the eye from high glucose levels.

MSM and Diabetes: Lack of sulphur can result in low insulin production. High blood sugar levels can be caused by poor cell permeability - glucose cannot enter the cell in optimum quantities for correct metabolism. Regular consumption of MSM can improve cell membrane permeability, the pancreas returns to normal as blood sugar is better absorbed through the cell walls, thus helping to balance blood sugar levels.

Chapter IXV

RESVERATROL AND DIABETES

Does This Plant Hold the Key to Controlling Diabetes

The grape extract known as **resveratrol** already has some **very** impressive accomplishments chalked up on its scoreboard. Also high up on that scoreboard are the extract's potential abilities to fight aging, cancer, inflammation, and Alzheimer's. And, of course, there are the mouse and rat studies that have hinted at resveratrol's ability to improve insulin sensitivity. (Well, in **rodents** at least.)

Now some exciting findings by Hungarian researchers from the University of Pécs are highlighting the compound's potential for reducing insulin resistance and fighting Type-II diabetes in humans.

After the four weeks, the scientists found that the people who had received the resveratrol had a **significant** decrease in their insulin resistance as compared with the placebo group. After eating a meal, both the time it took to reach the **maximum glucose level** and the extent of the **initial glucose drop**, were **significantly** different between the two groups with the resveratrol users being the clear winners

The researchers have a couple of theories about **how** the resveratrol is affecting insulin resistance. The first has to do with the compound's strong antioxidant abilities. Since oxidative stress plays a key role in insulin resistance, the resveratrol may be interrupting this process. The second theory has to do with resveratrol's ability to activate a specific protein…Akt phosphorylation…that's involved in your cells' ability to absorb glucose. The researchers observed an increase in the levels of this protein in those volunteers who took the resveratrol.

And the good news is that it's super easy to add more of it to your diet. The compound is found naturally in grapes, wine, grape juice, peanuts, blueberries, bilberries, and cranberries. Or, if you prefer, you can try a resveratrol supplement instead.

Reference: "Resveratrol improves insulin sensitivity, reduces oxidative stress and activates the Akt pathway in type 2 diabetic patients," **Br J Nutr**. 2011 Mar 9:1-7. [Epub ahead OF PRINT)

DIABETES RELATED TOPICS

Diabetic Foot Care

People with diabetes are prone to foot problems because of the likelihood of damage to blood vessels and nerves and a decreased ability to fight infection. Problems with blood flow and damage to nerves may cause an injury to the foot to go unnoticed until infection develops. Death of skin and other tissue can occur. If left untreated, the affected foot may need to be amputated. Diabetes is the most common condition leading to amputations.

To prevent injury to the feet, people with diabetes should adopt a daily routine of checking and caring for the feet as follows:Check feet every day, and report sores or changes and signs of infection

Wash feet every day with lukewarm water and mild soap, and dry them thoroughly.Soften dry skin with lotion or petroleum jelly.Protect feet with comfortable, well-fitting shoes.

Diabetics can use Foot Care Cream from www.pharmatech1.com

Exercise daily to promote good circulation.Remove shoes and socks during a visit to your health care provider and remind him or her to examine your feet.Stop smoking, which hinders blood flow to the feet

DIA CREAM AS EXTERNAL HEALING CREAM FOR DIABETES

*A number of diabetics used DIA CREAM on their **foot** and **umbilicus**, (also known as the **belly button**) twice daily and found big differences in their blood sugar readings.This experiment was done under the follow-up of Dr.B.Khasawneh.*

DEAD SEA BLACK MUD THERAPY FOR DIABETES

Diabetes patients can benefit from use of Mud Therapy, Mud Pack and Mud Bath. Mud therapy uses mud or clay packs, poultices and even mud baths to prevent, treat various diseases.

Chapter IXV

- It cools nervous system, activates different body organs and eliminates toxic matter from the body.
- Mud has several therapeutic qualities because it is rich in organic content.
- It takes longer to get heated and can hold the heat for a long time.
- The skin can tolerate mud at even high temperature.
- Compared to water bath, mud bath has milder action and is superior form of heat therapy.
- But mud loses its superior quality when it dries off.
- Mud used for mud treatment is preferably stored in tubs made of cast iron, wood, cement and ceramic.
- Two separate adjacent rooms are used for mud treatment.
- The room where mud is applied should have washable floors and walls.
- The mud is superheated before use.
- The room has also cold and hot water spray provision for washing after mud bath.
- The second room has a bed to rest after the bath. The same room can also be used for changing.

Mud bath increases circulation, tones and energizes the skin tissues.

The duration of the bath ranges from 30 minutes to 1 hour.

These therapeutic mud which is rich in natural minerals that enhance the production of enzymes in all living organisms provides 100% natural detoxification for Arsenic, Environmental, Aluminum, Dental Amalgam, Smoker's Drug, Copper & Lead, Mercury, Formaldehyde, Radiation and more. Technically, the mud first adsorbs toxins (heavy metals, free radicals, pesticides), attracting them to its extensive surface area where they adhere like flies to sticky paper; then it absorbs the toxins, taking them in the way a sponge mops up a kitchen counter mess. Clay's adsorptive and absorptive qualities may be the key

183

to its multifaceted healing abilities. Knishinsky reports(in hi that drinking mud or clay helped him eliminate painful ganglion cysts (tumors attached to jois book: the Clay Cure)nts and tendons, in his case, in his wrist) in two months, without surgery.

How To Prevent Gestational Diabetes

A new study has found that it is possible to prevent the onset of Gestational Diabetes in an expectant mother by making simple changes in the mother's diet. The study, done by researchers at UCSF(University of California - San Francisco), found that a chemical called serotonin influences the onset of Gestational Diabetes in an expectant mother. Since serotonin is made from the amino acid tryptophan which is found abundantly in high-protein foods, eating foods rich in protein during early pregnancy may prevent gestational diabetes in pregnant women.

How Does Serotonin Prevent Gestational Diabetes?

Pregnancy can cause several changes in the mother's metabolism. The energy requirements of the fetus are met by increased levels of insulin resistance in the mother's body. Since insulin is the hormone which carries glucose molecules in the blood to the molecular cells, insulin resistance causes the nutrients to be channeled in to the growing fetus instead of going to the mother's body. The mother's body counterbalances the insulin resistance and prevents hyperglycemia by the increased production of insulin-producing beta cells.

Serotonin, a chemical produced by the body and a known neurotransmitter, is the underlying agent that signals the stimulation of beta cell proliferation during the early pregnancy. Since serotonin is made from tryptophan - an amino acid that comes from high-protein foods such as milk, eggs, meat and fish - the study shows that increased intake of high-protein foods during the early pregnancy can cause higher production of serotonin and subsequently higher levels of insulin.According to UCSF Professor Michael German, MD, who is also the senior author of the paper, tryptophan hydroxylase (Tph1), the enzyme that produces serotonin from tryptophan increased by as much 1000-fold during the early pregnancy. The researchers found that inhibition of serotonin synthesis by restricting the intake of tryptophan in pregnant mice blocked beta cell proliferation and resulted in the development of glucose intolerance and gestational diabetes in the mice.

The research indicates that anything that affects the production of serotonin, such as drugs, diet or genetic inheritance may affect the risk of developing gestational diabetes and possibly the long-term risk of developing type 2 diabetes.

Serotonin has been widely studied as a neurotransmitter in the brain for its effects on appetite and mood, especially depression. Since it also influences the insulin production, this could explain why some patients with gestational diabetes experience depression. This would also explain the effect of some classes of psychiatric medications on diabetes.

The study will be published in the upcoming issue of "Nature Medicine" and was published online on June 27, 2010.

DIET AND DIABETES

Obese and overweight individuals suffering metabolic syndrome and Type 2 diabetes showed significant health improvements after only three weeks of diet and moderate exercise even though the participants remained overweight.

"The study shows, contrary to common belief, that Type 2 diabetes and metabolic syndrome can be reversed solely through lifestyle changes," according to lead researcher Christian Roberts of University of California, Los Angeles.

"This regimen reversed a clinical diagnosis of Type 2 diabetes or metabolic syndrome in about half the participants who had either of those conditions. However, the regimen may not have reversed damage such as plaque development in the arteries," Roberts said. "However, if Type 2 diabetes and metabolic syndrome continue to be controlled, further damage would likely be minimized and it's plausible that continuing to follow the program long-term may result in reversal of atherosclerosis."

"The results are all the more interesting because the changes occurred in the absence of major weight loss, challenging the commonly held belief that individuals must normalize their weight before achieving health benefits," Roberts said. Participants did lose two to three pounds per week, but they were still obese after the 3-week study.

The study involved 31 men who ate a high-fiber, low-fat diet with no limit to the number of calories they could consume. The participants also did 45-60 minutes of aerobic exercise per day on a treadmill.

Fifteen of the men had metabolic syndrome, a condition that is characterized by excessive abdominal fat, insulin resistance, and blood fat disorders such as high levels of triglycerides (fat in the blood) or low levels of HDL (high density lipoprotein, or "good" cholesterol). Thirteen of the participants had Type 2 diabetes. There was also some overlap between the two groups and some participants who had neither metabolic syndrome nor Type 2 diabetes, but were overweight or obese.

"The diet, combined with moderate exercise, improved many factors that contribute to heart disease and that are indirect measures of plaque progression in the arteries, including insulin resistance, high cholesterol, and markers of developing atherosclerosis," Roberts said. "The approach used in this experiment of combining exercise with a diet of unlimited calories is unusual."

Low-Calorie Foods

The participants in the current study, who ranged in age from 46 to 76 years old, took part in a 21-day residential program at the Pritikin Longevity Center, formerly in Santa Monica, combining the Pritikin diet and exercise program. The daily diet was low fat (12-15% of calories), moderate protein (15-20% of calories), and high in unrefined carbohydrates (65-70% of calories) and fiber (more than 40 grams).

PLANTS FOR DIABETES AND THEIR COMPOSITION

From Duke's Phytochemical Database here is a list of the most anti-diabetic and hypoglycemic herbs:

Number of Chemicals in Plants with Hypoglycemic Activity

Panax quinquefolius (Ginseng) Plant - 15 chemicals

Allium sativum var. sativum (Garlic) Bulb - 13 chemicals

Chapter IXV

Camellia sinensis (Tea) Leaf - 13 chemicals

Allium cepa (Onion) Bulb - 12 chemicals

Lycopersicon esculentum (Tomato) Fruit - 12 chemicals

Vitis vinifera (Grape) Fruit - 12 chemicals

Daucus carota (Carrot) Root - 11 chemicals

Foeniculum vulgare (Fennel) Fruit - 11 chemicals

Pisum sativum (Pea) Seed - 11 chemicals

Citrus paradisi (Grapefruit) Fruit - 10 chemicals

Musa x paradisiaca (Banana) Fruit - 10 chemicals

Achillea millefolium (Yarrow) Plant - 9 chemicals

Brassica oleracea var. botrytis l. var. botrytis (Cauliflower) Leaf -9 chemicals

Humulus lupulus (Hops) Fruit - 9 chemicals

Medicago sativa subsp. sativa (Alfalfa) Plant - 9 chemicals

Panax ginseng (Ginseng) Root - 9 chemicals

Ribes nigrum (Black Currant) Fruit - 9 chemicals

Solanum melongena (Eggplant) Fruit - 9 chemicals

Sorbus aucubaria (Rowan Berry) Fruit - 9 chemicals

Trigonella foenum-graecum (Fenugreek) Seed - 9 chemicals

Zea mays (Corn) Seed - 9 chemicals

Number of Chemicals in Plants with Antidiabetic Activity

Allium cepa (Onion) Bulb - 17 chemicals

Musa x paradisiaca (Banana) Fruit - 14 chemicals

Sorbus aucubaria (Rowan Berry) Fruit - 14 chemicals

Allium sativum var. sativum (Garlic) Bulb - 13 chemicals

Daucus carota (Carrot) Root - 13 chemicals

Humulus lupulus (Hops) Fruit - 13 chemicals

Lycopersicon esculentum (Tomato) Fruit - 13 chemicals

Vitis vinifera (Grape) Fruit - 13 chemicals

Camellia sinensis (Tea) Leaf - 12 chemicals

Pisum sativum (Pea) Seed - 12 chemicals

Ribes nigrum (Black Currant) Fruit - 12 chemicals

Citrus sinensis (Orange) Fruit - 11 chemicals

Foeniculum vulgare (Fennel) Fruit - 11 chemicals

Glycine max (Soybean) Seed - 11 chemicals

Hordeum vulgare (Barley) Seed - 11 chemicals

Medicago sativa subsp. sativa (Alfalfa) Plant - 11 chemicals

Panax quinquefolius (Ginseng) Plant - 11 chemicals

Ribes uva-crispa (Gooseberry) Fruit - 11 chemicals

Triticum aestivum (Wheat) Seed - 11 chemicals

Brassica oleracea var. botrytis l. var. botrytis (Cauliflower) Leaf -10 chemicals

Brassica oleracea var. capitata l. var. capitata (Cabbage) Leaf - 10 chemicals

NATURAL REMEDIES

Natural Cures For Diabetes (don't rely on any one remedy alone)

- I received this natural cure for diabetes from an Ayurvedic doctor who swears that anyone who follows it will be permanently cured of diabetes within two months. I know it sounds too good to be true, but it does deserve serious consideration, as she is a respected member in her field.

-Take 50 gm. of colocynth 50 gm. of acacia speciosa 50 gm of acacia arabica.

-Take these ingredients and crush and mix them up equally into a powder. Put into capsules, and take enough to equal two grams of the powder, once a day.

Chapter IXV

- Apple Cider Vinegar And Cinnamon: A very effective natural remedy for diabetes is to use apple cider vinegar and cinnamon. Take two tablespoons of raw unfiltered organic apple cider vinegar, mixed with four to six ounces of liquid and one teaspoon of cinnamon. (why not use green tea?)I take apple cider vinegar at least twice a day with a teaspoon of baking soda. The baking soda keeps the vinegar from hurting my teeth, and it's great for raising the bodies alkalinity. It's also fun to watch the vinegar fizz up. Either apple cider vinegar or cinnamon by themselves, are both reputed to be very effective natural cures for diabetes, but together? Well all I can say is, welcome to the wonderful world of holistic health and healing.

- DR. TONY ALMEIDA (Bombay Kidney Speciality expert) made the extensive experiments with perseverance and patience and discovered a successful treatment for diabetes.

Mix Ingredients:

 1 - Wheat flour 100 gm 2 - Gum(of tree) (gondh) 100 gm

3 -Barley 100 gm 4 - Black Seeds 100 gm

Method of Preparation Put all the above ingredients in 5 cups of water.

Boil it for 10 minutes and put off the fire. Allow it to cool down by itself.

When it has become cold, filter out the seeds and preserve the water in a glass jug or bottle..

How to use it?

Take one small cup of this water every day early morning when your stomach is empty.

Continue this for 7 days. Next week repeat the same but on alternate days. With these 2 weeks of treatment you will wonder to see that you have become normal and can eat normal food without problem.

Note: You can try it under your doctor supervision and do not leave your medication on sudden basis.

CHAPTER XX

DIABETES & ALKALINITY & ACIDITY
MEATS, BREAD AND CARBONATED BEVERAGES

The Herbal Insider Archives reported about how Acidity and Alkalinity affect human health as follows: (Scientists report that over 150 degenerative diseases are caused by high acid levels in the body). Knowing this fact, we should begin by understanding what acidity and alkalinity are and how they relate to our health.

The pH scale ranges from 0 to 14, with 0 being extremely acidic, 14 being extremely alkaline and 7 being neutral. Body fluids range between 4.5 and 7.5 pH (blood must maintain 7.35 to 7.45 pH). A one point drop on the pH scale is 10 times more acidic; for example from 7 to 6 is 10 times more acidic, from 7 to 5 is 100 times, from 7 to 2 is 1,000,000 times more acidic. Most plants and fish thrive in waters of pH values from 6.6 to 7.4. This is a good rule of thumb to use for humans as parasites, viruses, bad bacteria, and degenerative diseases are more prevalent in an acidic system. In order for the body to remain healthy, it keeps a delicate and precise balance of blood pH at 7.365, which is slightly alkaline. The body does whatever it has to in order to maintain this balance. The problem is that most people have incredibly acid-forming lifestyles. Acid is produced in your body whenever you have stress, upset emotions and when the food you eat is acid-forming.

The human body is composed of 78% water. The cells in the body are 98% water. Even our bones are 20% water. We can live for thirty days without food but only 3 days without water. If all the water is removed from a 150 pound person, the residue left would weigh less than 35 pounds. We know that the body fluids of healthy people are slightly alkaline while the same fluids of those who are sick are acidic, either very acidic or slightly. Generally speaking, the more acid your body is, the more serious the illness you have. The degree of acidity significantly affects the body's ability to prevent and/or reverse illness and disease (including such degenerative diseases as **cancer**, **diabetes**, heart disease, and others). Individuals that have severe health challenges almost invariably also have high acidity. Unfortunately, acidity has become a national epidemic that is one of the most ignored or unknown underlying causes of many of the degenerative diseases of the western world.

High systemic acid levels contribute or cause directly, numerous health problems;

- Acid systems can't use calcium effectively.

- They can't maintain proper blood oxygen levels and cancer can only develop in an oxygen poor, acidic environment.

- Acidic blood can't circulate properly creating extra strain on the heart.

- It adversely affects the digestive system and the lymphatic system.)

Basile Daskalakis wrote about the **effect of pH on diabetes**:

(Finally there is a proven system of pH balance diet and exercise that it will prevent, stop and reverse your Diabetes. Great health requires pH balance and you restore it with alkaline water and alkaline food

Our bodies work optimal in an alkaline fluids terrain. Alkalizing and alkaline foods will help you restore pH balance and get rid of acid wastes.

All the billions of cells that make up the human body are slightly alkaline ,and must maintain alkalinity in order to function and remain healthy and alive.

Alkaline foods are mostly green foods and vegetables, especially raw ones.

Some other healthy, alkaline foods are sunflower sprouts, flax oil, brown basmati rice, millet, soaked almonds, tomato slices, fresh avocado, vegetable soups or green vegetable juices.

All these foods offer a low carbohydrate, **high fiber** and delicious nutrition and a way to nourish your system with what it really needs to avoid the body cells to over-acidify.
Green grasses such as barley or wheat grass are some of the lowest-calorie, lowest-sugar and most nutrient-rich foods on earth, and contain high amounts of fiber.

Lemons and grapefruits are sour but alkaline.
A convenience food category includes chocolate, canned goods and fast food among the acidic foods. A balanced diet and proper exercise is naturally conducive to good bone health.

Many alkaline foods are natural choices for a healthy eating plan but they are not meant to treat or prevent any medical condition without guidance from a physician.

Chapter XX

All animal proteins, fats, sugars, soft drinks, coffee, vinegar are very acidic. Most green vegetable, fresh green juices, nuts, fresh fruits are alkaline in nature.

All those foods offer a low carbohydrate, high fiber and delicious nutrition and a way to nourish your system with what it really needs to avoid the body cells to over-acidify the main cause of diabetes 2.

By consuming alkaline foods and drinking alkaline water you restore your pH balance.

All the billions of cells that make up the human body are slightly alkaline see pH scale, and must maintain alkalinity in order to function and remain healthy and alive.

Alkaline food diet is a lifestyle based on eating foods that metabolize in an alkaline residue of minerals instead of acids. Result: What results you will actually get from an alkaline diet, within the first few days, weeks and months, depends on the severity of your diabetes and your lifestyle.

An imbalanced diet **high in acidic foods such as animal protein, sugar, caffeine**, and processed foods tends to disrupt this balance. It can deplete the body of alkaline minerals such as sodium, potassium, magnesium, and calcium, making people prone to chronic and degenerative disease.

Most doctors believe the healthy benefits of the alkaline diet. Who is this diet for? This diet is for people who feel unwell on a high fat, low carb diet. It is also for people who lead stressful lives and consume large amounts of acidifying foods such as protein, sugar, processed food, cereals, starches, and caffeine, with little alkalinizing vegetables.

Modern proponents of the alkaline diet look at the pH of blood, saliva, and urine, in addition to health symptoms and other factors. Since no disease or infection - including a fungal infection - can live in an alkaline state it is a good idea to keep the body close to its natural ph.

The alkaline diet is popular among people dieting for optimum health and safe weight loss.

However, most doctors agree that the alkaline diet is a good way to maintain general health.

Another benefit of following this diet is that the focus on eating high fiber, low fat meals will create a reduction in daily caloric intake.

The alkaline diet is easy to follow because it does not eliminate foods; Moderation is the golden rule. If you use moderation you can eat most of the foods.

This is also a simple diet because it is so adaptable.
The key to success when following any diet is planning meals in advance.
The Mayo Clinic Diet Manual lists the most alkaline fruits as dried figs, cantaloupe, watermelon, and dried apricots.

The list of alkaline vegetables includes: broccoli cabbage carrots cauliflower celery eggplant mushrooms squash turnips.
Acid foods should not be removed from your daily diet. On the alkaline diet they should be eaten in limited quantities, otherwise the alkaline level can become too high.

In general, it is important to eat a diet that contains foods from both sides of the chart.

The alkaline acid diet proposes that it is the acidity in food which causes our body to function sub-optimally.
Benefits of eating a healthier diet, like the acid alkaline diet include, potentially reducing the risk or severity of cardiovascular disease, cancer, obesity, diabetes, osteoporosis, gastrointestinal disease and acne.

Typical Western diets include too much of what are termed acid foods, in too high quantities.

Some highly alkaline fruit and vegetables include spinach, raisins and dried figs.

Eating so called acid foods is not a bad thing in itself. Rather it is eating a diet that contains too high a percentage of acidic foods that could become a problem.

The diet is based upon natural or holistic healing methods and has been around for quite some time.
Over eighty percent of one's food should comprise of fruits and vegetables if the normal slightly alkaline body ph. is to be maintained.
With an alkaline pH. your life span can be increased too. An alkaline diet is the best way to achieve acid alkaline ph. balance.
Besides hydrating the body with alkaline water, it is equally important to create the proper balance of alkaline and acid forming foods through a healthy alkaline diet.

Different sources offer conflicting information about foods suitable for an alkaline diet.

Chapter XX

Whether you consider adopting an alkaline diet for Crones disease or for optimal health benefits, it helps to explore your dietary options.

An alkaline diet lifestyle will make you feel alive and vital; The alkaline diet improves concentration,mental and physical stamina and overall self-esteem.

Thorough scientific studies are lacking on the alkaline diet. Most doctors believe the healthy benefits of the alkaline diet. Modern proponents of the alkaline diet look at the pH of blood, saliva, and urine, in addition to health symptoms and other factors. The alkaline diet is popular among people dieting for optimum health and safe weight loss.

However, most doctors agree that the alkaline diet is a good way to maintain general health.

Evidence supports that alkaline diets prevent kidney stones, osteoporosis, and muscle wasting disease due to aging. People who ascribe to the alkaline diet believe that eating foods leading to a high body acid content creates an imbalance of the normal acid and alkaline levels, and that this imbalance causes the loss of essential minerals from the body's system.

The alkaline diet is easy to follow because it does not eliminate foods; Moderation is the golden rule. If you use moderation you can eat most of the foods Knowing what types of foods are included in the alkaline diet will. allow you to plan meals ahead of time.

Some recommended fruits to be included in the alkaline diet: apples bananas blackberries dates On the alkaline diet they should be eaten in limited quantities, otherwise the alkaline level can become too high The acid alkaline diet attempts to show that there is a further nutritional benefit from fruit and vegetables, predominately. alkaline foods, which is the alkalizing effect they have upon us

Benefits of eating a healthier diet, like the acid alkaline diet include, potentially reducing the risk or severity of cardiovascular disease, cancer, obesity, diabetes, osteoporosis, gastrointestinal disease and acne.

Alkaline diet supporters believe the body uses essential minerals such as calcium and potassium to neutralize acid and maintain a healthy ph.

Testing your pH;

Test your body's pH before deciding if an alkaline diet might help

195

you.

Dr. M Ted Morter Jr, M A, author of "Your Health, Your Choice," says that an alkaline diet will replenish whatever minerals you use to neutralize acid.

I decided to put together an alkaline diet chart to display what food are considered to be alkaline and healthful and which ones are considered acidic and should be avoided!

Conclusion:
Alkaline diet eliminates the main causes of diabetes. It is the best diet in preventing diabetes in the first place. Make a choice and stay healthy with an alkaline diet lifestyle. It will be a lot harder to reverse diabetes than prevent diabetes.)

We can find full details of the effect of Ph on diabetes in **Dr.Robert Young: The pH Miracle for Diabetes: The Revolutionary Diet Plan for Type 1 and Type 2 Diabetics.**

Effect of Meat Consumption on Diabetes and Health

Dr. Morse, wrote in his book: *The Detox Miracle Sourcebook:*

Protein from meat is highly acid-forming, lowering the body's pH balance. This causes inflammation and tissue weakness, leading to tissue death. • When protein breaks down, it creates sulfuric and phosphoric acids, which are highly irritating, inflammatory, toxic and damaging to tissue. These acids also stimulate nerve responses leading to hyperactivity of tissues.

• Because of the high acidic content, too much meat protein has also been linked to colon cancer, the second largest type of cancer in America today. Thousands of people die each year from the accumulated effects of eating high protein diets. The liver, pancreas, kidneys and intestines are destroyed when protein consumption is too high

• Protein is a nitrogen compound, high in phosphorous, which when consumed in large amounts, will deplete calcium and other electrolytes from the body.

• Some of the final digestive states of protein-matter result in the production of uric acid. Uric acid is abrasive and irritating, which inflames and damages tissues. Uric acid deposits can create arthritis in the joints and muscle tissue. Uric acid causes gout.

Effect of Carbonated Beverages on Diabetes and Health

Chapter XX

As per studies conducted **carbonated** beverages are most **acidic** drinks amongst all .The most famous and popular soft drinks are highly acidic ; their pH values range between 2.5 and 3.0 However, this fact is not given much of publicity as it can affect the business of several companies. Acid can never have a good effect on your stomach. It is a complete myth that carbonated beverages can treat an upset stomach. Also carbonated beverages are high on sugars, calories and other additives that can prove harmful for your stomach. As per research conducted, it has been proved that intake of carbonated beverages can cause osteoporosis which is a disease of bones, these drinks can also cause irritation in your stomach, and hasten the decay your teeth. Carbonated drinks absorb calcium from the blood, depriving you of the same. Some beverages are also high on salt that can cause dehydration.

Too much of carbonated beverages results in cell mutation that can pose a high risk. These drinks can also result in obesity, as it is high on calories.

Too much carbonated beverages can prove fatal in the near future and it is best to stay away from them. Juices and water are better sources to quench thirst and also get some vitamins and nutrients. So the next time you feel thirsty, try out a glass of juice or water and feel the difference.

From:ScienceDaily (Aug. 23, 2007) — Researchers have found new evidence that soft drinks sweetened with high-fructose corn syrup (HFCS) may contribute to the development of diabetes, particularly in children. In a laboratory study of commonly consumed carbonated beverages, the scientists found that drinks containing the syrup had high levels of reactive compounds that have been shown by others to have the potential to trigger cell and tissue damage that could cause the disease, which is at epidemic levels.

Be Aware of Diet Drinks

Since diet soda drinks are sweetened with the sweet chemical poison;aspartame it is much safer to drink regular drinks because of the 92 dangers caused by consuming aspartame sweetener.For more information please read Chapter 13 of this book.

Alkaline Healthy Water

Ionized Water is Alkaline

Because it is very Alkaline, Ionized Water dissolves accumulated

197

acid waste and returns the body to a proper pH balance. Just by supplying your daily drinking and cooking water from a Water Ionizer, you can restore a healthy alkaline environment in your body.

Ionized Water is a Powerful Antioxidant

Imagine having the ability to take normal tap water and turn it into an antioxidant with a negative ORP, which retards the aging process. Millions are spent each year on antioxidizing vitamins such as Vitamin C and E, and enzymes. Yet a glass of alkaline water has **more antioxidant power than orange juice!** Anti-oxidants prevent cellular and DNA damage by neutralizing free radicals! Of all other types of water commonly available today, ONLY alkaline ionized water (also known as "reduced" water) is strongly antioxidizing.

The Killer in White Bread and White Flour

Did you know...that **White bread is very acidic**

Chlorine gas, potassium bromate are used to remove any slight yellow color (bleach) wheat flour to make it white. But in the process, a by-product called **alloxan** is created that actually **destroys** beta cells in the pancreas responsible for making insulin!

Scientists regularly use alloxan to induce diabetes in lab animals because it destroys the insulin-producing function of the pancreas, allowing glucose levels to shoot sky-high.

Consuming white flour products has the same effect on your blood sugar as eating table sugar! And it also damages your pancreas.

In the manufacture of white flour ; 6 layers of seed bran are removed ,and the germ which contains 76% of vitamins and minerals,97% of fiber are lost!!! It is further bleached with harmful chemicals .It is further whitened by chalk,alum and aluminuim carbonate.Some studies showed that Lab rats die in 7-10 days when placed on white flour!!!!

CHAPTER XXI

DIABETES AND GLUTEN-FREE DIET

From American Diabetes Association:

(Gluten is a protein found in wheat, rye, barley and all foods that are made with these grains.

Celiac disease is a digestive disorder. When someone with celiac disease eats food containing gluten, their body reacts by damaging the small intestine. Uncomfortable symptoms such as abdominal pain often occur. The damage to the small intestine also interferes with the body's ability to make use of the nutrients in food.

About 1% of the total population has celiac disease. It is more common in people with type 1 diabetes. An estimated 10% of people with type 1 also have celiac.

The only way to manage celiac disease is to completely avoid all foods that have gluten. Following a gluten-free diet will prevent permanent damage to your body and will help you feel better.

Gluten Intolerance

There are also many people who are said to have a gluten intolerance. When these people eat foods that contain gluten, they also experience uncomfortable symptoms. However, they test negative for celiac disease and actual damage to their small intestine does not occur. More research about gluten intolerance is needed, but avoiding foods with gluten should help to relieve these symptoms).

New England Journal of Medicine listed 155 diseases linked to gluten !!! One of those is diabetes I & II.

The most dangerous gluten-containing food that should be avoided by diabetics is white flour. You can read more details about it in Chapter 20 of this book.

Treating Diabetes with Gluten-Free Diet

(From: *diabetichealthtoday.com)*

(Diabetics most definitely benefit from a gluten-free diet . This type of diet is a way of life for people suffering from diabetes as well as other diseases such as celiac, autism and many other diseases.

Dr. Mansour

Many people especially diabetics have severe gluten sensitivities. Many illnesses have been associated with gluten consumption and one out of every hundred has gluten intolerance. People that suffer from infections such as diabetics develop this type of sensitivity.

Eating gluten-free diet has helped people not only with Type 1 and Type 2 diabetesbut also diseases like celiac, multiple sclerosis, rheumatoid arthritis, and inflammation of the nervous system, peripheral neuropathies, anaemia, seizures and loss of balance.

What is a gluten-free diet? Foods that contain gluten such as wheat, oats, rye, barley, pasta, cereal, beer and spelt should be avoided. Many processed foods also contain gluten. One can buy bread and pastas that are gluten-free as well as many other products which can be obtained from most supermarkets and health outlets. All fresh fruits and vegetables are gluten-free as well as potato, rice, soy, and buckwheat and bean flour.

Farmers that grow grain increase the amount of gluten in their products because grain having a higher protein content fetches a higher market price. However companies are aware of the fact that many people suffer from gluten intolerance are improving the taste of gluten-free products. Those that suffer from gluten in tolerances can also opt for integrative manual therapy which helps with physical pain and loss of function as in diabetics as well as change their diet to gluten-free diet as it has been noted recently that there is a gluten sensitivity epidemic.

It has also been noted that those with gluten sensitivity have deficiencies in manganese, zinc and chlorophyll as well as smooth and skeletal muscle weakness which are linked to the large intestine and gluten. A gluten-free diet will improve one's health all round and also ensures that more nutrients will reach areas that have already been damaged and will also help stabilize blood sugar levels in diabetics.

There have been positive results and diabetics have reported back that their symptoms were alleviated after a few weeks when they changed to a gluten-free diet. However it is important to remember that a diabetic patient should first discuss any and all diet plan with their primary medical practitioner or dietitian.)

One of the best gluten-free bread are sorghum and millet bread . The good nes is that we have arrived this year to produce a 100% gluten-free bread, biscuit, pasta and chips from sorghum and millet by using a 2 herbal binding agents

CHAPTER XXII
DIABETES AND SPORTS
Blood Flow Circulation

It is well known that diabetes of both types causes blood flow insufficiency throughout the whole body.

All types of of sports including walking on daily basis do improve blood circulation.Moreover sports is essential for the provision of oxygen and nutrients to all the cells of the body – for both living and healing

Enhancing blood flow inside leg and foot accelerates wound healing and prevents diabetic foot gangrene.

Burning Calories & Better Control of Blood Glucose:

When a diabetic starts with an exercise program or one is an athlete, he is already aware that he should pay closer attention to his diet and monitor his blood glucose more frequently. This is a more effective key to control and reduce complications of diabetes.

The most important sports that diabetic can benefit to burn calories and lower his/her sugar are the following:

Jogging: At a speed of 6 km/h, in 30 minutes, the human body consumes over 450 calories meaning the same that we accumulate by eating 85 g of chocolate. Jogging has important positive effects on respirator and cardiovascular device. It is important for you to be properly dressed up taking into consideration that while jogging we sweat a lot. The footwear must also be adequate to avoid any accident.

Mountain hiking: This is a sport that shouldn't be done without out of hand preparation. Articulation mobility is very important as by mountain hiking we lose over 370 calories in 30 minutes. Be careful to the equipment and to the specified rules concerning this sport. Read about it before practicing.

Swimming: It is true what is said: swimming is a very complex sport which brings benefits to all the body and favors consonant development to bone and muscles. By swimming for half an hour, we consume over 360 calories. If 30 minutes swimming is too much you can, take a pause.

Cycle: At a speed of 30 km/h the organism burns over 350 calories in 30 minutes. So just a bike walk isn't enough. You just make an effort. Cycling favors muscles development and has benefic effect on circulatory apparatus and on the heart. Take into consideration also the fact that cycling has the benefits of a comfortable travel.

This sport is recommended to those who have some kilos in advantage as the weight is being taken over by the bicycle, not by your own legs.

Boxing: Women doing boxing is no longer a strange thing. Sometimes you feel the need of a brutal release, isn't it? 30 minutes of boxing helps you eliminate 325 calories. Do you want to know other boxing benefits? It entrenches the cardiopulmonary system, pectoral, arms and leg muscles.

In conclusion try doing as much sport as you can! It will surely make you feel great and burn calories and sugar daily.

Sports Increase Insulin Sensitivity:

The exercising diabetics may experience increased glucose uptake at a given insulin concentration. Exercise does not promote more production of insulin, but it increases insulin sensitivity by enhancing receptor site biding. This effect can persist for several hours, up to 24 hours in some individuals. Due to it, non-insulin dependent diabetics may be able to reduce doses of medication (oral hypoglycemic medications or insulin). Reducing insulin levels, the diabetic become more protect from atherosclerotic damages.

Reduction in Blood Pressure:

The reduction of blood pressure is another benefit from exercise. Loss of weight and decreased stress, which are the consequences of sports/exercise are recognized as safe factors for diabetics.

Heart Disease and Stroke.

Daily sports can help prevent heart disease and stroke by strengthening heart muscle, lowering blood pressure, raising high-density lipoprotein (HDL) levels (good cholesterol) and lowering low-density lipoprotein (LDL) levels (bad cholesterol), improving blood flow, and increasing heart's working capacity.

Chapter XXII

Sports Reduce Stress ,Depression and Tension

It is well known that sports reduce stress that often leads to increased blood sugar.

Sports Reduce Obesity

Obesity. Sports help to reduce body fat by building or preserving muscle mass and improving the body's ability to use calories. When sports are combined with proper nutrition, it can help control weight and prevent obesity, which is a major risk factor for diabetes .

Sport and hypoglycemia

Physical activity can cause hypoglycemia in two differing ways. Blood sugars can go low during exercise and sugar levels can also drop several hours after. Different people respond differently to activity. Therefore kids with type I diabetes should be cautious during sports sessions.

CHAPTER XXIII

DIABETES AND DEPRESSION

P.J.Lustma et al in a recent study published by Diabetes Care Journal said:

Depression in diabetes is a prevalent and chronic condition. The etiology is unknown but is probably complex; and biological, genetic, and psychological factors remain as potential contributors. Several neuroendocrine and neurotransmitter abnormalities common to both depression and diabetes have been identified, adding to etiological speculations. Pharmacotherapy of depression may improve both mood and glucose regulation in diabetes, although controlled studies of the efficacy of psychotherapy and pharmacotherapy for depression in diabetes are not yet available. Depression has potential interactions with diabetes on multiple levels and remains an important clinical focus independent of the medical disease.

In another study published in the same journal W.W.Eaton et al concluded that:

Major depressive disorder signals increased risk for onset of type II diabetes.

Diabetes and depression form a deadly combination, increasing the risk of death according to a study published in the same journal.

The study found that people who have the combination of type 2 diabetes and minor depression have a 67% greater risk of dying. While people with both diabetes and major depression have a 130% greater chance of dying, compared to those who have type 2 diabetes alone.

A recent University of California study showed that people having a depressing day were more likely than people in a good mood to report higher blood sugar .

In fact if you have diabetes your chances of also having depression are twice as likely as some who does not have diabetes.

How is Depression and Diabetes Linked?

Depression increases stress and hypertension the thing which affect release of insulin which is strongly inhibited by the stress   hormone norepinephrine (noradrenaline), which leads to increased blood glucose levels during stress.

Depression can directly influence specific physiological body processes that can make diabetes worse. These include immune responses, inflammation and even insulin resistance.

Whatever comes first, diabetes and depression are related and have become the focus of many researchers. Your focus on good health and overall well- being will help you in your fight against diabetes and depression.

How do you know if you suffer from depression?. If you have five or more of the following symptoms :

- persistent sadness ,feeling of hopelessness,feelings of guilt, worthlessness, or helplessness,loss of interest or pleasure in hobbies, decreased energy, fatigue , difficulty concentrating and making decisions insomnia or oversleeping , appetite changes, restlessness, irritability, thoughts of death or suicide(if you have this one , even if it's the only symptom, please get immediate help.

Don't allow depression and diabetes to defeat you.

Use the combination of a natural diabetes formula together with our aromatherapy **RELAX U PERFUME** and our easy program to help you in your fight against diabetes and depression

CHAPTER IXXV

PROF.MANSOUR STRATEGIC PROTOCOL TO LOWER BLOOD SUGAR FROM 400 TO 100 NATURALLY

Our protocol to reverse diabetes and lower sugar from 400 to less than 100 on permanent basis without medications is as follows:

DIABETES I & II
(Beneficial Remedies, Treatments, and Nutrients)

HERBAL COMBINATIONS: DIA TECH 2000,GLUCO LIFE and Similar Dietary Supplements

SINGLE HERB : Alfalfa,Aloe Vera, Banaba, Basil, Bilberry, Bitter Melon, Buchu, Cat's Claw, Cayenne, Ceder Berries, Cinnamon, Coriander, Fenugreek Seed, Flax Seed, Garlic, Ginkgo Biloba, Evening Primrose Oil, Ginseng, Glucomannan, Goat's Rue, Goldenseal, Gymnema Sylvestre,Nettle,Licorice Root,Milk Thistle, Neem, Olive Leaf, Figs Leaf, Pau D'Arco, Mullein, Stevia, Suma, Sumac, Rehmania, Juniper and Uva Ursi.

VITAMINS: A, B complex, B1, Benfotiamine, B2, B6, B12, Choline, Inositol ,Taurine, D3, E, K2 and P.

MINERALS: Calcium, Chromium, Iron, Potassium, Phosphorous, Manganese, Magnesium, Selenium, Vanadium, and Zinc.

ALSO: Alpha Lipoic Acid,Beta Glucan (From Barley, Shiitake, Maitake, Reishi Mushrooms, or Flax Seed) Brewr's, Yeast, Biotin, CQ10, Lecithin, Fiber, Protein, FishOil, MSM, Arabinoxylan, Celluluse, Arabic Gum, and Benfotiamine

AMINO ACIDS:L- Carnitine, N-Acetyl Cysteine, Glutathione, Arginine

HERBAL TEAS: Tetohuxtle Tea,Green Tea,Black Tea,Essiac Tea, Dia Tea (Cassia Arriculata Tea), Milagro de la , Selva tea, Ginger/Mate tea.

DRINKS AND JUICES: *Camel Milk* (Natural Insulin), Lemon Juice/Ginger and Vinegar, Mangosteen juice, Grapefruit Juice, Aloe Vera Juice ,Noni Juice,Blueberry Juice,Cranberry Juice, Pomegranate

Juice,Alfalfa Juice,Yogurt,Vegetable Juices. Nopal Extract juice to lower blood sugar as well as to regulate cholesterol levels and inflammation of the liver, hepatitis. Wheat grass juice has proven to be beneficial for diabetes, Cholesterol,Cancer, Aids, Skin Disorders, Kidney Liver ,Colon, High Blood Pressure and Immunity, Barley grass, and Goji Juice.

CREAMS: DIA CREAM,FOOT CREAM

SOUPS: Cream of Broccoli,Ginger Curry Carrot soup,Asparagus soup, Lentil soup,Spiced Pumpkin soup, Clam Chowder soup **,Radish-Celery-Cinnamon-Ginger-Onion-Garlic soup.**

SALAD: Daily salad of green leaves, parsley, onion, garlic, sunflower oil,apple cider vinegar

BATH: Dead Sea Black Mud Therapy.

SPORTS: Walking for 30 minutes daily, Swimming and Cycling.

HELPFUL FOODS: **Almond,**Apricots, Artichoke, Asparagus, bananas, beef, **celery** juice,chicken, blackstrap molasses, butter, cheese, lentils, kidney beans,oysters, carrots, turnip greens, and soybeans.

AVOID: ASPARTAME & ALL DIET FOOD & DRINKS which contain Aspartame, Smoking, Wine, Saturated fatty acids.

DIABETIC FOOT GANGRENE PROTOCOL

SPECIFICS: Gangrene is the reduced or stopped blood flow which results in oxygen deprived tissue. It may be caused by frostbite, poor circulation, hardening of the arteries, diabetes, or could be the result of a wound or injury.

(Beneficial Remedies, Treatments, and Nutrients)

SINGLE HERBS: Barberry, Basil,Red Pepper,Black Cohosh, Cayenne, Echinacea,Ginger, Ginkgo Biloba, Golden Seal, Kelp,Marshmallow, Rosemary,and Licorice.

VITAMINS: Multi-vitamin plus A, C, and E.

MINERALS: Calcium, Magnesium, Potassium, and Zinc.

CREAMS: Foot Cream 3 times daily.

ULTRASOUND THERAPY: High Intensity Focused Ultrasound (HIFU) twice daily.

ALSO: DMG, Coenzyme QIO, Germanium, and Proteolytic enzymes.

HELPFUL FOODS: Apples, bananas, citrus fruits, broccoli, carrots, green and green leafy vegetables, cheese, herring, oysters, fish liver oils, and aloe Vera.

CHAPTER XXV

FACTORS THAT DELAY CURE (IS THERE A CURE FOR DIABETES?)

Prof.Mansour Essential Information for Diabetics:

Guidelines & Golden Tips to Arrive at the Port of Cure

1-Take Moderate Light Meals, Small amounts of sweets & avoid dates.

2-Try to take 4 to 5 snack meals daily and avoid heavy meals.

3-Avoid White Bread and eat Whole Wheat Bread

4- Avoid Butter, Margarine, Trans fats, also called partially hydrogenated oils and use Olive Oil,Cocunut Oil and Jojoba oil only.

5-Try to walk or swim for 30 minutes per day.

6-Eat plenty of Garlic and Onion with or without low fat Yogurt..

7-Eat Organic Cucumber,Squash,Gourd and Zucchini

8-Drink a tea composed of fenugreek and cinnamon on daily basis

9- Drink a Tea of Ginseng-Green Tea-Ginger on frequent basis..

10-Add Apple Cider Vinegar to your daily green salad.

11-Cut 2 Okra fingers into pieces and infuse them in a cup of water over night and drink it in the morning.

12-Use diet high in fiber further helps to stabilize blood sugar by slowing the absorption of carbohydrates and supports a healthy lower bowel and digestive tract. Try to gradually increase fiber to 30 to 50 grams a day..

13-Drink Camel Milk(natural insulin) if available.

14-Try to use botanical herbal drug for diabetes and consult your doctor.

15-Take Vitamin D3 together with your herbal medications

16- Take Propolis or Azithromycin to fight any infection.

17- Increase number of Kisses with your lovely partner on daily basis.

18-Perform sex with your lovely partner 3 times per week or more.

19- Keep your blood pressure under control.

20- Have enough time of sleep in night time and do not reverse day and night.

21-Read or listen Quran/Holy books and listen to music on daily basis.

22.Use Aromatherapy oil like RELAX U PERFUME on forehead with gentle massage frequently.

23- Use Dia Cream or foot cream on foot with gentle massage..

24-Measure your fasting blood sugar and post prandial on daily basis and tabulate all results.Test your HbA1c every 3 months.

What Delays Cure from Diabetes?

1-Presence of H.Pylori in your stomach.

2-Any viral or bacterial infection in any part of the body ; flu, urinary, prostate, bone,...will close the Islets cells partially or totally and raise insulin resistance and delay sugar burning!!

3- Any Stress or Nervous shock closes iselet cells too... Be always calm.

4-Thyroid disorder.

5- Irritible Bowel Syndrome(Colon)

6-High Bad Cholesterol (LDL).

7- Smoking causes venous insufficiency and lipid deposits.

8- Metformin causes venous insufficiency,stroke and renal failure

9-Avandia causes liver cirrhosis.

10-Aspartame and artificial sweeteners cause 92 diseases including 2 types of cancers. Please see   www.dorway.net

11- Lack of sleep .

12- Lack of sex.

CHAPTER XXVI

THE ROLE OF MARINE PHYTOPLANKTON IN DIABETES

What is Marine Phytoplankton?

Marine Phytoplankton is a single-celled aquatic organism, or micro-algae. It is not a plant, seaweed, fungus or herb. Thousands of species of phytoplankton grow abundantly in oceans around the world and are the foundation of the marine food chain.

Marine Phytoplankton can be described as "The Jewel Of The Ocean". It contains a unique combination of life-sustaining nutrients and antioxidants including: essential fatty acids, amino acids, protein, vitamins, chlorophyll, minerals, trace elements, & phytonutrients.

Marine Phytoplankton may be the most nutrient dense food on Earth. The primitive character of this micro-algae's cellular structure gives it a number of advantages over higher plants and animals as a food source. Nearly the entire organism is nutritious, with minimal indigestible structures. By contrast, typically less than half the dry weight of raw fruit and vegetables have any nutrient value.

According to NASA, Marine Phytoplankton produces about 90% of the Oxygen in the air that we breathe. Marine Phytoplankton also absorbs most of the Carbon Dioxide in the atmosphere, helping to mantain a balanced ecosystem which is essential for a healthy planet.

More than 99% of all creatures that live in the ocean depend either directly or indirectly on Marine Phytoplankton for their survival. Thanks to this micro-algae, some species of Whale can enjoy an active and reproductive life for up to 200 years.

In the wild, Marine Phytoplankton is invisible to the naked eye. However, under certain conditions this micro-algae can be seen from a space satellite.

Marine Phytoplankton exhibits superior photosynthetic efficiency, using light approximately three times more efficiently than higher plants. Micro-algae are among the most productive organisms on the planet.

The blue whale is king of the seas. It's diet consists of marine phytoplankton and a species of krill which, also eat phytoplankton. The blue whale can travel hundreds of miles without rest.

Phytoplankton have an **alkaline pH**. Many diets are high in refined sugars, soda pop, and farmed large animals which cause the body to be in a state of acidity. Alkaline foods are necessary to balance the body's ph.

Here is a just a small sample of health conditions that Ocean's Alive can be used for:

Obesity -- help boost metabolism and give cells more energy, thereby facilitating weight loss

Memory Loss -- break through the Blood Brain Barrier, thereby reaching the deepest glands in the brain, which can help to stimulate neurotransmitter production and increase brain function and memory

Diabetes -- alleviate mineral deficiency in the bloodstream, thereby helping to restore normal glucose levels.

Faster Healing Time -- accelerate cellular repair, thereby enabling the body to heal itself more rapidly

* Neurological Disorders -- deliver important nervous-system repair agents such as phospholipids, DHA and EPA, thereby helping to reconstruct the protective sheathing around nerve cells, which rejuvenates them.

Fatigue -- provide more oxygen to cells, thereby boosting energy levels and alleviating tiredness and fatigue

Poor Eyesight -- its high antioxidant content helps improve eyesight.

Also Phytoplankton contains a unique combination of life sustaining nutrients including; Omega 3 essential fatty acids (EPA and DHA), protein, chlorophyll, vitamins, minerals and trace elements., Marine Phytoplankton reduces the levels of sugar in the bloodstream of the diabetic patient. The most reknown feature of Marine Phytoplankton as one of the natural cures for diabetes is that it **not only improves the blood sugar levels, but it also prevents the usual complications that arise from diabetes**. Testimonials show dramatic changes in glucose

Chapter XXVI

levels of those who choose to use marine phytoplankton, although it must already be established as one's maintenance intake for diabetics because losing the supply of marine phytoplankton may spike glucose levels at abnormal levels again.

Type I, or Juvenile Diabetes, is defined by the pancreas losing its ability to produce insulin. It is more severe than Type II, which is characterized by insulin resistance at the cell membrane level. Inflammation, oxidation, mitochondrial dysfunction, and toxicity of the cell membrane result in pancreatic dysfunction, and insulin resistance in each cell of our bodies, thereby explaining the problems seen with both types of diabetes. Marine phytoplankton can help restore function to the cell by correcting those issues with its high content of antioxidants, anti-inflammatory nutrients, and its ability to enhance detoxification pathways in the liver, intestines, kidneys and skin; energy-producing pathways in the mitochondria are also enhanced.

Marine phytoplankton's nutrients improve our immune system in the intestines and in the body, thereby minimizing the damage that our immune system may bring to the pancreas and cell membranes throughout our body. Marine phytoplankton reduces the amount of sugar present in our bloodstream, thereby reducing the myriad of complications seen in diabetics (eye problems, ulcers in extremities, heart disease, strokes, hormone problems, neurologic and immune system dysfunction, etc.).

Some people worry that the transient elevation of blood sugar noted while consuming fruits in general, is a sign that these foods are not good for diabetics. As noted on the front cover of the March 2005 issue of the Journal Neuron, this reasoning is not justified. In fact, this very misconception leaves people to lack antioxidants that are essential to build and fuel their cell membranes. Furthermore, they end up dissatisfied and craving sugar in general and refined foods

CHAPTER XXVII
POSSIBLE CURES FOR TYPE I DIABETES

Researchers find possible cure for type 1 diabetes

Posted by Jimmy Hibsch at 9:53 p.m., Feb. 4, 2011

Researchers at the University of Texas Southwestern Medical Center might have found a possible cure for type 1 diabetes, converting it to a asymptomatic, non-insulin-dependent disorder.

"We've all been brought up to think insulin is the all-powerful hormone without which life is impossible, but that isn't the case," said Roger Unger, professor of internal medicine and senior author of the study appearing online and in the February issue of Diabetes in a news release. "If diabetes is defined as restoration of glucose homeostasis to normal, then this treatment can perhaps be considered very close to a 'cure.'"

Studies on mice show that when glucagon, a hormone produced by the pancreas, is suppressed, insulin becomes completely unnecessary. The hormone's absence does not cause diabetes or any other abnormalities, according to the release.

Normally, glucagon prevents low blood sugar levels. In individuals with type 1 diabetes however, it causes high blood sugar.

Type 1 diabetes affects about one million people in the United States.

Friendly Bacteria Protect Against Type 1 Diabetes

In a dramatic illustration of the potential for microbes to prevent disease, researchers have shown that mice exposed to common stomach bacteria are protected against the development of type 1 diabetes.

The findings support the "hygiene hypothesis" -- the theory that a lack of exposure to parasites, bacteria and viruses in the developed world may lead to increased risk of diseases like allergies, asthma, and other disorders of the immune system.

The results also suggest that exposure to some forms of bacteria might actually help prevent onset of type 1 diabetes, which is an autoimmune disease. In Type I diabetes, the patient's immune system launches an attack on cells in the pancreas that produce insulin.

CHAPTER XXVIII

ARE STEM CELLS A POSSIBLE CURE FOR TYPE I DIABETES?

By JUNKO TAKESHITA ABC News Medical Unit -April 10, 2007

An injection of stem cells could one day serve as a therapy for diabetes, a new study suggests, demonstrating yet another application for the versatile stem cell approach.

In the current issue of the Journal of the American Medical Association, a small Brazilian study reports that injections of stem cells harvested from a patient's own blood may keep type 1 diabetes at bay. The type 1 form of diabetes accounts for 5 to 10 percent of the approximately 21 million Americans with the disease.

The injections work by using the patient's own stem cells to replace the defective cells that cause the disease.

The study's findings could bring new hope to patients with type 1 diabetes because "for the first time in the history of diabetes, patients are now treatment-free for up to three years," says Dr. Richard Burt, the senior author of the study and chief of the division of immunotherapy at Northwestern University's Feinberg School of Medicine.

But some diabetes experts say more research is needed to confirm the benefits.

Dr. Jay Skyler, associate director of the Diabetes Research Institute in Miami and author of an accompanying editorial to the study, cautions that the study "is pioneering and provocative, but it is too small a number and too short a duration to allow people yet to change. ... It needs confirmation."

And since the treatment involves destroying the patient's immune system before the patient receives the stem cells, critics fear the risks of the treatment may outweigh its potential benefits.

When Immune Cells Attack

Type 1 diabetes is caused by the destruction of the insulin-producing cells in the pancreas by a person's own immune cells -- what Burt calls the "police force" of the body.

The disease is usually diagnosed in childhood or adolescence. Patients normally face a lifelong regimen of insulin replacement, either through a continuous pump or frequent self-administered insulin shots.

Insulin is critical to how the body uses sugar. Without it, unused sugar, or glucose, builds up in the body.

Over the long term, chronically high levels of glucose can damage the eyes, heart, kidneys and nerves -- possibly resulting in blindness, heart disease, kidney failure and loss of sensation.

Currently, there is no cure for type 1 diabetes, and only strict control of glucose levels can reduce the complications of this disease. But Burt and his colleagues hope that these stem cell injections could be a first step.

Though this is the first time researchers have used this particular stem cell approach for diabetes, such injections have been found to be promising in the treatment of many other diseases in which the immune system attacks the patient's own body, such as rheumatoid arthritis and multiple sclerosis.

First, doctors collect the patient's own stem cells from his or her blood. They then destroy the patient's existing immune cells with chemicals, after which they use the harvested stem cells to rebuild the patient's immune system.

Unlike the old immune cells, the new ones will not attack the insulin-producing cells in the pancreas or at least, that's what researchers hope.

Too Little, Too Early

But is this study good enough? Skyler cautions that the research is limited by three things: small numbers, short duration and no control group.

Our Observations and Comments

We met a number of our friends who did stem cells in a famous center in Germany and they informed us that they felt good for 5 months only and their blood sugar became worse than before in the sixth month.They were asked to repeat it and they did and after another 6 month their status became worse.

218

CHAPTER IXXX

THE HEALING POWER OF OZONE AND H2O2

Adult –Onset Diabetes – Oxygenated Blood Can Help

From: Alternative Medicine Magazine,Issue 26, November 1998; Pages 26-28

YOU DON'T normally think of oxygen as a treatment for diabetes, but according to Frank Shallenberger, M.D., H.M.D., director of the Nevada Center of Alternative and Anti-Aging Medicine in Carson City, Nevada, ozone (a less stable, more reactive form of oxygen) can produce remarkable improvements in both the major and secondary symptoms of adult- onset diabetes. The connection between the ozone and diabetes is the blood circulation, Dr. Shallenberger says, as demonstrated in the following cases.

Virginia, 51, had been diabetic for five years and was taking Glucotrol, an oral medication for controlling blood sugar levels. However, Virginia came to Dr. Shallenberger seeking treatment for recurrent breast cancer, a tumor that periodically grew then diminished.

Dr. Shallenberger decided to ozonate her blood as ozone is often used as a healing substance in alternative cancer treatments. He drew 150 cc of Virginia's blood then injected it with ozone gas. Ozonating the sample of Virginia's blood took about 40 minutes, after which it was re infused into her body. He did this daily to address the cancer.

What surprised Dr. Shallenberger in this case was that not only the breast cancer responded to ozonation (it started to dissolve) but so did Virginia's diabetes. Her blood sugar levels began dropping too low (a condition called hypoglycemia) indicating that the ozone and Glucotrol were controlling her blood sugar too well. Dr. Shallenberger reduced her Glucotrol dosage to once daily, then soon after, as the low blood sugar trend continued, eliminated the drug altogether. "Practically speaking, Virginia didn't have diabetes any longer," notes Dr. Shallenberger.

How did ozone bring her diabetes under control? Diabetics always run the risk of complications, such as loss of vision, heart disease, nerve dysfunction, and gangrenous limbs. Diabetics usually have considerable circulation problems such that the actual blood flow to their tissues is diminished, explains Dr. Shallenberger. Patients often have difficulty digesting fats (such as cholesterol and triglycerides) and their arteries tend to thicken and harden.

"This is compounded by the fact that what little blood reaches their tissues is less effective than it should be and is unable to deliver oxygen to those tissues," says Dr. Shallenberger. "The tissues become oxygen depleted, which explains why diabetics have problems with gangrene and why they're unable to resist infections."

A prime reason the red blood cells in the diabetic's blood are unable to release their oxygen is that a key molecule called 2,3-diphosphoglycerate, or 2,3-dpg for short, is in reduced supply. Under normal conditions, 2,3-dpg stimulates red blood cells which carry oxygen to deliver it to the tissues; but if there isn't enough of this molecule in the system, the red blood cells can't deliver the oxygen.

When you introduce ozone--that is, more oxygen-into the blood, more 2,3-dpg is produced and the oxygen-delivery system and the efficiency of blood circulation start to improve. The ozone also appears to enhance the activity of cellular metabolism, the continual conversion of food into energy. Dr. Shallenberger likens the metabolism-heightening effect of ozone to a similar benefit to diabetics obtained through vigorous exercise. It oxygenates the tissues and gets all the body processes running better, he says.

Levels of ATP, an important molecule which stores energy in the cells, are also enhanced through ozonation. Among other functions, ATP helps each cell maintain the integrity of its membrane, thereby enabling it to regulate the passage of materials into and out of the cell, says Dr. Shallenberger. If the cell membrane collapses, the cell dies; if a lot of cells die you start getting tissue death, and gangrene becomes a possibility.

Gangrene in a toe was a serious diabetic complication besetting Quentin, 50. His diabetes was poorly controlled, mainly because he was reluctant to comply with dietary restrictions, says Dr. Shallenberger.

Quentin's blood sugar level was around 230; a safe, normal level ranges between 70 and 120.

Dr. Shallenberger already had worked with Quentin for two years, prescribing dietary changes, herbs, and supplements, but when Quentin developed gangrene on the third toe of his right foot and conventional

Chapter IXXX ────────────────

doctors were scheduling him for amputation at the ankle, Dr. Shallenberger decided to try ozonation. "Quentin's toe was completely black and they were going to amputate his entire foot because the rest of the tissue was on the borderline of becoming gangrenous, too," he notes.

For Quentin's treatment, Dr. Shallenberger added another element to the ozonation procedure: chelation. The Chelation would help improve Quentin's blood circulation by removing heavy metals and arterial plaque. Dr. Shallenberger calls his combined treatment "chezone."

Chelation improves blood circulation to the tissues, he explains, which means they get more oxygen. This in turn improves their metabolic rate (energy processing efficiency) and enables them to make better use of glucose (blood sugar). When you have higher efficiency in using glucose, you are much closer to controlling the diabetes naturally, says Dr. Shallenberger. Using ozone, as stated above, helps the patient utilize the available oxygen better, due to improved circulation. Combining Chelation with ozone in effect doubles the circulation benefits.

In addition to chezone, Dr. Shallenberger put an ozone extremity bag around Quentin's right foot, filled it with ozone gas, and left it in place for 20 minutes. In this way, the ozone was absorbed through the skin, an approach that has proven successful in treating chronic sores and skin ulcers, says Dr. Shallenberger.

Each time he gave Quentin a chezone treatment (ten in all, one per day), he also ozonated his foot. After about two weeks, the foot was much improved; the area between the ankle and gangrenous toe had healed which meant only the toe would have to be amputated.

After the surgery, Quentin hurt his foot in such a way that the stitches broke open and a large ulcerating sore formed. His doctors talked about amputation again, but after another six weeks of chezone and foot ozonation treatments, Quentin's foot healed again. Following the first two weeks of intensive treatments, Dr. Shallenberger gave him a chezone once weekly and foot ozonation three times weekly. In ensuing months, Quentin received maintenance treatments.

About ten weeks after the first chezone treatment, "the lesion in Quentin's foot was entirely healed and he was down to only two Micronase pills a day," says Dr. Shallenberger. "If I had been able to treat his toe before it went black, I probably could have saved it." As it turned out, Dr. Shallenberger did save Quentin's right foot twice.

In the case of Leonard, 64, controlling his sugar intake was central to being able to get his diabetes and gangrene complications under control. Leonard, who developed diabetes six years earlier, was on insulin and Glucophage (another diabetes drug) to control his blood sugar levels.

However, Leonard developed a blister on the sole of his foot; when this became infected, his doctor cleaned out all the infected tissue, leaving a hole in his foot. Over a three-month period, this wound failed to heal even with antibiotics and Leonard's doctors were talking about amputating his foot.

Dr. Shallenberger started Leonard on the same combination chezone and foot ozonation program that had worked so well for Quentin. Then he added a piece of advice. "You must cut down on your sugar intake." Leonard ate a lot of white sugar in his diet and none of his conventional doctors apparently made the link between high dietary sugar intake and the inability of his infection to heal. "White blood cells, the immune cells that fight infection, cease to function in the presence of elevated glucose levels," says Dr. Shallenberger.

After two treatments, Leonard's foot was noticeably improved and his energy levels were heightened. The initial progress motivated Leonard to comply fully with the program. Dr. Shallenberger started Leonard on a series of nutrients and remedies including chromium and vanadium, to help his body utilize its natural pancreatic insulin.

People with adult-onset diabetes produce insulin but their system becomes unable to use it, a condition called insulin resistance. In fact, the pancreas of such a patient generally produces too much insulin; as the body fails to act on this insulin, the pancreas produces yet more. The minerals chromium and vanadium break this cycle and support the body in making use again of pancreatic insulin, says Dr. Shallenberger.

Among the other elements of Leonard's program were pancreatic enzymes (to support pancreas function and to improve digestion; 400-800 mg three times daily), the hormone melatonin (to bolster the immune system; 3 mg once daily), and the hormone DHEA, levels of which tend to be about 50% below normal in diabetics.

Low DHEA levels may help explain the characteristic weight gain in people with adult-onset diabetes, says Dr. Shallenberger. He notes that DHEA doses will vary with each patient. "Women should take enough (usually 10-25 mg daily) to raise the serum DHEA-sulfate to between 2,000 and 3,000 mg/ml, while men should take enough (usually 50-100 mg daily) to raise it to between 3,000 and 4,000 mg/ml."

He also gave Leonard a specialized product (made from the fungus Mucor racemosus) called Mucokehl, developed in Germany by the

Chapter IXXX

Sanum company, and now used selectively (as part of a line of several dozen similar substances) by North American physicians. The Mucokehl would help regulate microorganisms which affect the thickness and texture of the blood.

After a month of treatments, Leonard's foot was completely healed, says Dr. Shallenberger. As his blood sugar came under better control, Leonard was able to lower his daily insulin intake and resume his busy life.

Hydrogen Peroxide for Diabetes

Hydrogen peroxide is a clear, colorless liquid that easily mixes with water. It is a compound made up of two hydrogen atoms and two oxygen atoms and is known chemically as $H2O2$. Hydrogen peroxide is created in the atmosphere when ultraviolet light strikes oxygen in the presence of moisture. Ozone ($O3$) is free oxygen (O) plus an extra atom of oxygen. When it comes into contact with water, this extra atom of oxygen splits off very easily. Water ($H2O$) combines with the extra atom of oxygen and becomes hydrogen peroxide ($H2O2$).

We can call hydrogen peroxide a close relative of ozone. Aside from being known as a powerful oxygenator and oxidizer, a special quality of hydrogen peroxide is its ability to readily decompose into water and oxygen. Like ozone, hydrogen peroxide reacts easily with other substances and is able to kill bacteria, fungi, parasites, viruses, and some types of tumor cells.

Hydrogen peroxide occurs naturally within the Earth's biosphere; traces of it are found in rain and snow. It has also been found in many of the healing springs of the world, including Fatima in Portugal, Lourdes in France, and the Shrine of St. Anne in Quebec. Hydrogen peroxide is an important component of plant life, and small amounts are found in many vegetables and fruits, including fresh cabbage, tomatoes, asparagus, green peppers, watercress, oranges, apples, and watermelons.

Hydrogen peroxide is also found in the animal kingdom and is involved in many of our body's natural processes. As an oxygenator, it is able to deliver small quantities of oxygen to the blood and other vital systems throughout the body. Hydrogen peroxide does not oxygenate the body merely by producing modest amounts of oxygen, however; it has an extraordinary capacity to stimulate oxidative enzymes, which have the ability to change the chemical component of other substances (like viruses and bacteria) without being changed themselves. Rather than providing more oxygen to the cells, the presence of hydrogen peroxide enhances natural cellular oxidative processes, which increases the body's ability to use what oxygen is available.

Hydrogen peroxide must be present for our immune system to function properly. The cells in the body that fight infection (the class of white blood cells known as granulocytes) produce hydrogen peroxide as a first line of defense against harmful parasites, bacteria, viruses, and fungi. Hydrogen peroxide is also needed for the metabolism of protein, carbohydrates, fats, vitamins, and minerals. It is a by-product of cell metabolism (that is actively broken down by peroxidase), a hormonal regulator, and a necessary part of the body's production of estrogen, progesterone, and thyroxin. If that weren't enough, hydrogen peroxide is involved in the regulation of blood sugar and the production of energy in body cells

Hydrogen peroxide was discovered in 1818 by the French chemist Louis-Jacques Thenard, who named it eau oxygenee, or "oxygenated water." It has been used commercially since the mid-1800s as a nonpolluting bleaching agent, oxidizing agent, and disinfectant.

Effect of H2O2 On the Heart and Circulatory System
Hydrogen peroxide can dilate (expand) blood vessels in the heart, the extremities, the brain, and the lungs. It is also able to decrease heart rate, increase stroke volume (the amount of blood pumped by the left ventricle of the heart at each beat), and decrease vascular resistance (which makes it easier for blood to move through the blood vessels). As a result, it can increase total cardiac output.

Effect of H2O2 On Sugar (glucose) Utilization
Hydrogen peroxide is said to mimic the effects of insulin and has been used successfully to stabilize cases of diabetes mellitus type II

USING 35% FOOD GRADE HYDROGEN PEROXIDE (H202) - INTERNAL

It is suggested to take the below dosages either one hour before eating or 3 hours after eating.

Use the dosages listed in the chart with 5 ounces of distilled or purified water. When reaching higher dosages,more water may be used. Take on an empty stomach, 1 hour before a meal and at least 3 hours after a meal. If your stomach gets upset at any level, stay at that level, or go back one level. NOTE: Candida victims may need to start at 1 drop 3 times per day.

Chapter IXXX ━━━━━━━━━━━━━━━

Dosage Schedule for undiluted 35% H202
1st   day,use 9 drops (3 drops, 3 times/day)
2nd day,use 12 drops (4 drops, 3 times/day)
3rd   day,use 15 drops (5 drops, 3 times/day)
4th   day,use 18 drops (6 drops, 3 times/day)
5th   day,use 21 drops (7 drops, 3 times/day)
6th   day,use 24 drops (8 drops, 3 times/day)
7th   day,use 27 drops (9 drops, 3 times/day)
8th   day,use 30 drops (10 drops, 3 times/day)
9th   day,use 36 drops (12 drops, 3 times/day
10th day,use 42 drops (14 drops, 3 times/day)
11th day,use 48 drops (16 drops, 3 times/day)
12th day,use 54 drops (18 drops, 3 times/day
13th day,use 60 drops (20 drops, 3 times/day)
14th day,use 66 drops (22 drops, 3 times/day)
15th day,use 72 drops (24 drops, 3 times/day
16th day,use 75 drops (25 drops, 3 times/day)
For more serious complaints stay at 25 drops, 3 times per day for 1 - 3 weeks. Next graduate down to 25 drops, 2 times per day until the problem is taken care of. This may take from 1 - 6 months. Don't give up!
When free of complaints, you may taper off by taking:
25 drops once every other day, 4 times
25 drops once every third day for 2 weeks
25 drops once every fourth day for 3 weeks
A good maintenance would be 5 - 15 drops per week, depending on the amount of cooked and processed foods you are eating.

ALTERNATIVE METHODS

For those who have a tolerance problem with hydrogen peroxide, there are aloe vera mixtures available in several flavors that are quite palatable. These mixtures are taken undiluted, according to directions on the label.

Two such products are Super Oxy Plus Aloe Vera Tonic or Oxy Toddy. Many distributors stock these products or they may ordered from R.E.A.C.H., 4096 Bonita Road, Bonita, CA 91902., (619) 475-2874.

Intravenous Injections

Hydrogen peroxide is now being used intravenously and intra-arterially by a number of doctors in both the United States and in many foreign countries. The International Bio-Oxidative Medicine Foundation is supporting clinical research in this area. For doctor referrals, you may

Dr. Mansour

write or call: P.O. Box 13205, Oklahoma City, OK 73113, (405) 478-4266. (The usual donation is $5.00 if there is a doctor in your area.)

Dr. Kurt Donsbach uses hydrogen peroxide intravenously at Hospital Santa Monica at Rosarito Beach, Mexico. For information about the clinic and modalities used, call (619) 428-1147 or 1-800-359-6547.

SAFETY AND STORAGE TIPS FOR HYDROGEN PEROXIDE :Accidents can occur with hydrogen peroxide concentrate when safety precautions are not taken and directions are not followed. For this reason, we want to stress some safety and storage tips. Read them carefully and review the way you handle the concentrate to determine whether changes must be made with your handling procedure.

1. Keep hydrogen peroxide concentrate out of the reach of children.

2. Never transfer the concentrate into unlabeled or improperly labeled containers.

3. If hydrogen peroxide concentrate is accidentally spilled on the skin, flush the area immediately with running water.

4. If hydrogen peroxide concentrate is accidentally ingested, drink large amounts of water to dilute. Stay upright and contact your doctor. It could be toxic or fatal if swallowed at full strength.5. For spillage of hydrogen peroxide concentrate, dispose of according to Federal, State and local regulations.

Flush the spill area with water. Do not return the spilled material to the original container. Prevent undiluted hydrogen peroxide from entering into the sewage system. Report spills in compliance with Federal, State or local regulations.

Large quantities, such as drums, should be stored in a cool, dry area. When concentrations of hydrogen peroxide come in contact with organic materials, this may form explosive mixtures (spontaneous combustion).

Small quantities of 35% food grade hydrogen peroxide should be stored in the freezer over-wrapped with black plastic and labeled as to contents. Thirty-five percent food grade hydrogen peroxide will not freeze unless the temperature is 33 degrees below zero.

Low concentrations, such as 3% or 6% would freeze, so freezer storage is not recommended. Store properly labeled containers in a cool, dry place out of the reach of children.

CHAPTER XXX

How Enzymes Hold the Key to a Diabetes Cure
The Most Effective Natural Diabetes Treatments Plan?

Posted by Diabetes Cure: Enzymes Can hold the secret to diabetes cure? Doctors are not able to reject claims of diabetic cure with enzyme therapy because research has proven that it works wonders and accomplish successful results that normal medicines could never do

What is it anyway? Insulin is basically an enzyme that is secreted by the pancreas. The pancreas also secretes other digestive enzymes. Under diabetic conditions, the insulin level is reduced below the normal level. This is because of improper functioning of pancreas. So it is not just insulin, the level of other digestive enzymes are also drastically reduced.

What happens when the enzymes are reduced, anyway?

- Enzymes are the metabolic force of our body. When enzymes are reduced, the whole biological process of the body screeches to a halt. When enzymes are reduced, the body loses its basic functions and its immunity.

- Reduction in digestive enzymes results in accumulation of undigested proteins in the body. The proteins get accumulated in the kidney and result in major kidney failure.

- Enzymes are the catalyst for absorption of vitamins and minerals. Without enzymes, vitamins and minerals get accumulated without getting absorbed causing dangerous problems.

Enzyme therapy through natural diet supplements the body with the deficient enzymes to give the magic cure for diabetes

When you consume fully processed food containing processed grains, high fat content (we are talking about the bad fat and not the good one that helps the body), it does 2 things to the body:

- Digestive enzymes cannot act on the food that is highly processed. So when the nutrients do not reach the cells, they start to wear out.

- The body never accepts any unnatural intake. This results in the formation of toxins.

But don't worry. With selected natural dietary suggestion, you can improve the enzyme levels in the body and yes! You are back on track!!

Bob D Williams has been involved in the SEO field for over ten years. Working in various SEO services but specializing in link building services, professional custom videos and more.

How Enzymes Hold the Key for a Effective Natural Diabetes Treatments Cure ?

Important Enzymes:

For type 2 diabetes patients who have circulatory problems, it is important to take an enzyme supplement to help treat the symptoms of type 2 diabetes.

While the above treatment will cure your diabetes, you may have more immediate needs related to the side-effects of having diabetes.

Type 2 diabetes can be cured!! But before understanding any cure for type 2 diabetes, it is first necessary to understand the cause of type 2 diabetes.

First of all, **being overweight does NOT cause type 2 diabetes!!!** Scientists generate a lot of data, but frequently have **no clue** how to interpret the data.

The reason there is a high statistical correlation between being overweight and having type 2 diabetes is that the same thing that causes type 2 diabetes also causes some people to be overweight. For example, bad fats (such as in margarine) are what cause type 2 diabetes, and bad fats can also cause a person to be overweight.

Thus the statistical correlation is not a "causal" relationship, but rather a "common cause" relationship. It is extremely rare when a scientist discusses "common cause" statistical correlations because they get paid to sell drugs. **Let us repeat: being overweight does NOT cause type 2 diabetes.**

Here is more information about what really causes type 2 diabetes:

228

Chapter XXX

- *"Another lipid in a cell wall is cholesterol. And you thought it was a terrible thing. The cholesterol in each one of your cells forms a "hydrophobic" bond within the cell wall. Hydrophobic means "fear of water." It's a cute way to describe this function of our cells, but in our lives it simply describes the reason we don't melt in a rainstorm or fall apart when we take a shower or bath. Our cells resist water. Without this resistance, we would be water-soluble and we'd all dissolve in a rainstorm.*

  Our diets in this country (and in Budwig's country (Germany) at the time) lack these highly unsaturated fatty acids and contain an excess of man-made oils known as trans fats (or partially hydrogenated oils). These oils are very much like cholesterol and our bodies cannot tell the difference. These oils get into our cell walls and destroy the electrical charge. Without the charge, our cells start to suffocate. Without the oxygen, the only way the cell can replicate is anaerobically. (They also are very tough oils and have a 20-year shelf life. They impede the process of cellular exchange, or letting nutrition in and letting wastes out. Trans fats are also responsible for Type II diabetes, since insulin is a very large molecule it has a difficult time passing through a cell wall created with man-made fats and not cholesterol.)"
  http://www.mnwelldir.org/docs/cancer1/budwig.htm

In other words, trans-fatty acids attach themselves to the cell walls, and because they are a different type and shape of molecule, make the cell walls "rigid," and the large glucose molecules cannot penetrate the cell walls and get into the cells.

Here is a more detailed way to explain it (taken from an email from a medical doctor):

- *"Insulin binds with a cell wall receptor that causes a transport molecule to come to the wall and escort the glucose/ascorbate to where it is needed. The trouble is that it can't easily come through a port made of the wrong fatty acids. The cell may still have some good ports so increasing insulin will still help. Over time as the body continues to store excess glucose as triglyceride in fat cells and doesn't burn fat the person becomes obese--just look around you, it's everywhere.*

229

- *Most diets are low-fat and the fats they do contain are bad fats and the problem just gets worse."*

Type II or Type 2 diabetes is one of the rare diseases that is not caused by a microbe or impurities in vaccinations. It is caused by our diet of "bad fats" and the lack of "good fats" in our diet.

These same bad fats cause heart disease and many cases of people being overweight.

In other words, the same bad fats cause three major health problems:

1) Type 2 diabetes,

2) heart disease,

3) many cases of being overweight.

There are many other things these molecules cause as well.

The medical community, having no interest in what causes disease, claims that type 2 diabetes causes heart disease. This is partly true, but most of their statistical correlation is caused by the fact that both of them are caused by the same thing - the ratio of bad fats to good fats.

If a person were to simply avoid the trans-fatty acids and many other bad fats, eventually their type 2 diabetes would go away because as the bad cells (i.e. the ones with rigid fats on them) died, they would be replaced by new cells made of good fats (assuming there were good fats in your diet). However, this process would take several years since many cells live for multiple years.

However, there is a way to speed up the process. By avoiding the bad fats, and flooding your body with the right type of good fats, especially water-soluable omega 3, *type 2 diabetes is very easy to cure.*

It generally takes 7-12 months (much less time if it is newly diagnosed).

It is absolutely critical to avoid all trans-fatty acids , all hydrogenated oils,all canola oil,all margarine and all other bad fats because they are a plague on humanity!!

Scientists believe they are one step closer to finding a cure for Type 1 diabetes. Researchers believe they may be able to reverse Type 1 diabetes by blocking a newly identified enzyme that destroys beta cells in the pancreas that produce insulin.

A team of physicians at Eastern Virginia Medical School's Strelitz Diabetes Center have been able to identify the enzyme 12-Lipoxygenase (12-LO) as the culprit for Type 1 diabetes. The research group is one of the few able to receive help from individuals who have donated their bodies to science through the Juvenile Diabetes Research Foundation Islet Resource Center Consortium.

By studying human beta cells the scientists have discovered that 12-LO is an inflammatory enzyme that produces specific lipids that destroy beta cells. When beta cells in the pancreas are destroyed the organ no long produces insulin, leading to Type 1 diabetes. Blood sugar levels rise and lead to serious health consequences unless treatment is initiated.

Studies have shown that deleting the gene that produces 12-LO can stop Type 1 diabetes in mice. Studies of donated human beta cells have allowed the researchers to confirm that the enzyme is the cause of beta cell destruction from inflammation. "We've now confirmed that 12-LO is a relevant target in humans, particularly in the pancreas, and will help lead to new therapies," says the EVMS researchers.

The team is working with investigators in California and the National Institutes of Health to find medications that would target 12-LO as a new treatment that could stop the damage to beta cells that occurs in Type 1 diabetes. The researchers hope their findings will lead to a cure for Type 1 diabetes. (Journal of Clinical Endocrinology & Metabolism , doi: 10.1210/jo. 2009-2011).

An Alternative Safe Herbal Solution:

Gymnema Sylvestre: Restoration of Pancreatic Beta Cells
by: JoAnn Guest

May 22, 2003 11:59 PDT

GYMNEMA SYLVESTRE

Gymnema Sylvestre (family Asclepiadaceae) is a woody climber that grows in tropical forests of the central and southern parts of India, it has been used as a treatment for diabetes mellitus since ancient times.

The first scientific confirmation of this traditional use in human diabetics came almost 70 years ago when it was demonstrated that the leaves of GS reduced urine glucose in diabetics.

Four years later it was shown that GS had a blood glucose lowering effect when there was residual pancreatic function, but was without effect on animals lacking pancreatic function, suggesting a direct

effect on the pancreas.

EVIDENCE OF A MIRACLE

In 1990 a series of published studies on Gymnema Sylvestre Extract lifted this herb from interesting to revolutionary.

To begin with, it was shown that the administration of Gymnema Sylvestre Extract to diabetic animals not only resulted in improved glucose homeostasis, this improvement was accompanied by

regeneration of beta cells in the pancreas.

In the words of the authors, " This herbal therapy appears to bring about blood glucose homeostasis through increased serum insulin levels provided by repair/regeneration of the endocrine pancreas.

" To my knowledge, this is the only compound that has shown the ability to lessen indicators of diabetes by directly repairing/regenerating the pancreas cells responsible for producing insulin. As abnormalities in beta cell number and/or function are directly related to both Type I (insulin dependent) and Type II diabetes mellitus, it appeared that GS and Gymnema Sylvestre Extract was a major discovery in the battle against one of the most common disorders in the world.

Also in 1990, this same research team published results on their treatment of both Type I and Type II diaetics and Gymnema Sylvestre Extract over a period of more than 2 years.

In the case if Type II diabetics, Gymnema Sylvestre Extract resulted in significant reductions in blood glucose, glycosylated hemoglobin, glycosylated plasma proteins, and conventional drug dosage.

At the beginning of the study all participants were taking oral antidiabetic medication, and treatment with Gymnema Sylvestre Extract resulted not only in a lowering of oral medication necessity, but almost

Chapter XXX

25% of the participants were able to discontinue conventional oral medication and maintain blood glucose homeostasis with Gymnema Sylvestre Extract alone. Additionally,Gymnema Sylvestre Extract significantly improved cholesterol,triglyceride, and free fatty acid level's that were elevated in the study participants.

According to Dr. Baskaran and Dr. Ahamath, of the Department of Biochemistry, Post-Graduate Institute of Basic Medical Sciences,Madras, India, the therapeutic properties of Gymnema Sylvestre, an extract from the leaves of Gymnema Sylvestre, in controlling hyperglycaemia was investigated in 22 Type II diabetic patients on conventional oral anti-hyperglycaemic agents.

Gymnema Sylvestre, 400 mg/day) was administered for 18-20 months as a supplement to the conventional oral drugs.During Gymnema Sylvestre supplementation, the patients showed a significant reduction in blood glucose, glycosylated haemolglobin and glycosylated plasma proteins, and conventional drug dosage could be decreased.

Five of the 22 diabetic patients were able to discontinue their conventional drug and maintain their blood glucose homeostasis with Gymnema Sylvestre alone.These data suggest that the beta cells may be regenerated/repaire in Type II diabetic patients on Gymnema Sylvestre supplementation.

This is supported by the appearance of raised insulin levels in the serum of patients after Gymnema Sylvestre supplementation.

*Journal of Ethnopharmacology 1990;30; 295-300

Many of our Type I diabetics who took our food supplements which include gymnema sylvestre left insulin for good for more than 8 years and their tests showed normal HbA1C and C-Peptide values which validate healthy pancreas beta cells with healthy sugar levels!!

Dr. Mansour

Chapter XXX ────────────

About the Author

Awad Mansour, Ph.D.

Professor of Chemical Engineering & Pharmaceutical Industry
profmansour@gmail.com   www.pharmatech1.com
www.magicperfume.net
www.yarmouktourcure.com www.profmansour.com
www.swineflu-cures.com

PERSONAL : *D.O.B : March, 13, 1951*

EDUCATION : *B.Sc. in Chemical Engineering, Baghdad University 1975, M.Sc. & Ph.D. in Chemical Engineering, University of Tulsa, Oklahoma,U.S.A., 1980.*

TEACHING EXPERIENCE:1980-2008 with Yarmouk ,Jordan University of Science & Technology.
1993-1994 : University of Akron,Ohio,U.S.A. Chairman of of Chemical Engineering & Pharmaceutical
Department at Jordan University of Science & Technology 1989-1990.

PUBLICATIONS:*100 PUBLISHED PAPERS IN REFEREED JOURNALS*
PATENTS IN POLYMER, WATER & OIL INDUSTRY:
A Carry-Along Toilet "CARRYLET" a joint author with A.B. Shahalam M.O., Othman **registered in JORDAN, No. 87-1307, 1987.**,Multi-Purpose *Surfactant/Detergent for Oil Recovery from Water, Oil Spills, Tar Sands, Beach Sand and Shale Oil, Drag Reduction and Emulsification Processes, Kansas, (GemTech Solvents 1983-93),*
A New Drag Reducing Additive for Crude Oil Pipelines & Sanitary Sewers, Certified by the University of Akron, Ohio, U.S.A 1983-1995,A New Heat Reducing Additive for District Heating, HV AC Systems and Hydro-Power Plants, High Tech Technology, Cleveland & University of Akron, Akron, Ohio, U.S.A. 1993-1995.
A New Cold Technology for Shale Oil Extraction at Room Temperature,2006,
A New Surfactant to Separate Oil from Canadian Oil Sand at Room Temperature,. Edmonton, Alberta, Canada, 2006,New Surfactants to Solve Oil Spill Problems on Beaches and in the Sea, Certified by Alberta Research,Edmonton, Canada ,2001.
New Polymer Composites, Case Western & Reserve University, Cleveland, Ohio,

U.S.A. (1993-1994).A NEW Cold Biodiesel Production Using A New Efficient Technolgy; JORDA, 2008,New Nano Water Elecrolysis to Produce Commercial Hydrogen; Jordan,2008,New Ultrasonic Water Elecrolysis to Produce Commercial Hydrogen; Jordan,2008,New Nano Double Strength Concrete; JORDAN, 2009,A New Efficient Motor Oil Additive, JORDAN,2008.

PATENTS IN HERBAL MEDICINE
PRESS TECH: For Hypertension,AZMA TECH for Asthma.DIA TECH 2000: for Diabetes I & II. RENO TECH 2000: The First Cure for Kidney Failure. MG10,MG20 : for Cancer. IMU TECH&IMUFAST : for HIV, Hepatitis C & B. SPLEENO TECH for Spleen,VIA TECH: for Sex,PSORIA. TECH, LIV TECH, CHOLES TECH , PROSTA TECH,MC10 for malaria,JOINT TECH,RELAX U

CHEM. ENG. & COMPUTER BOOKS: *DRAG & HEAT REDUCTION, HTT, Ohio. U.S.A. 1995,AMAZON.COM*
Chemical Separation,ed. J.C..King,U.S.A.,Chapter on Adsorption.217-237(1986)
60 COMPUTER BOOKS: Published 1983-2008

HEALTH & MEDICINAL BOOKS:
DO NOT BE AFRAID OF SWINE FLU,AMAZON.COM,2009
The 50 Miracle Cures of Coriander, AMAZON.COM,2009
The 50 Miracle Cures of Curcumin, Health Tech Book Series,2009
60 HEALTH BOOKS ARE COMING IN U.S.A.

MEMBERSHIP IN SCIENTIFIC AND PROFESSIONAL SOCIETIES

- American Institute of Chemical Engineers and Jordanian Engineers' Society.
- AMERICAN HERB RESEARCH FOUNDATION
- AMERICAN HEALTH SCIENCES INSTITUTE
- INTERNATIONAL SOCIETY OH PHARMACEUTICAL ENGINEERING
- NEW YORK ACADEMY OF SCIENCES